IT'S
NOT
ABOUT
THE
BIKE

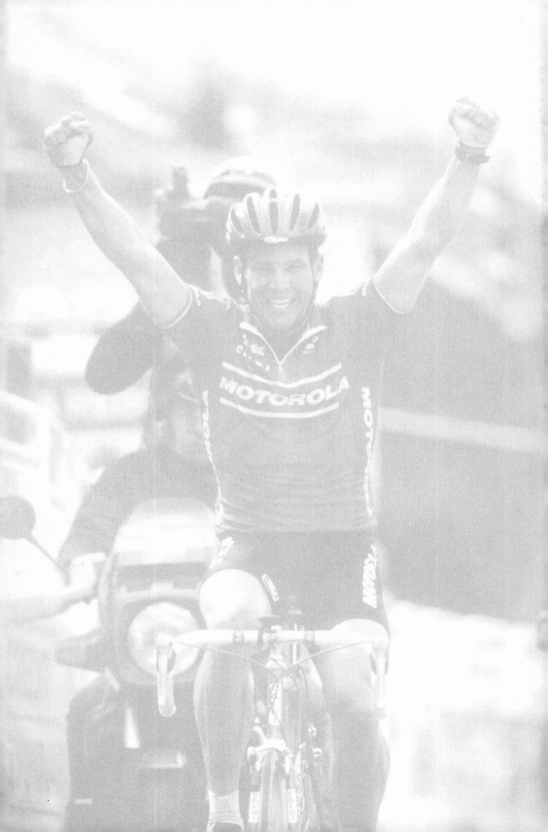

IT'S NOT ABOUT THE BIKE

My Journey Back to Life

LANCE ARMSTRONG

with Sally Jenkins

G. P. PUTNAM'S SONS ○ NEW YORK

G. P. Putnam's Sons
Publishers Since 1838
a member of
Penguin Putnam Inc.
375 Hudson Street
New York, NY 10014

Library of Congress Cataloging-in-Publication Data

Armstrong, Lance.
    It's not about the bike : my journey back to life /
Lance Armstrong with Sally Jenkins.
        p.   cm.
    ISBN 0-399-14611-3
    1. Armstrong, Lance.   2. Cyclists—United States—Biography.   3. Cancer
patients—United States—Biography.   I. Jenkins, Sally.   II. Title.
GV1051.A76 A3   2000   00-035612
796.6'2'092—dc21

Printed in the United States of America
10   9   8   7   6

This book is printed on acid-free paper. ∞

BOOK DESIGN BY AMANDA DEWEY
TITLE PAGE FRONTISPIECE BY GRAHAM WATSON

THIS BOOK IS FOR:

My mother, Linda, who showed me
    what a true champion is.
Kik, for completing me as a man.
Luke, the greatest gift of my life, who in a split second
    made the Tour de France seem very small.
All of my doctors and nurses.
Jim Ochowicz, for the fritters . . . every day.
My teammates, Kevin, Frankie, Tyler,
    George, and Christian.
Johan Bruyneel.
My sponsors.
Chris Carmichael.
Bill Stapleton for always being there.
Steve Wolff, my advocate.
Bart Knaggs, a man's man.
JT Neal, the toughest patient cancer has ever seen.
Kelly Davidson, a very special little lady.
Thom Weisel.
The Jeff Garvey family.
The entire staff of the Lance Armstrong Foundation.
The cities of Austin, Boone, Santa Barbara, and Nice.
Sally Jenkins—we met to write a book but
    you became a dear friend along the way.

The authors would like to thank Bill Stapleton of Capital Sports Ventures and Esther Newberg of ICM for sensing what a good match we would be and bringing us together on this book. Stacy Creamer of Putnam was a careful and caring editor and Stuart Calderwood provided valuable editorial advice and made everything right. We're grateful to ABC Sports for the comprehensive set of highlights, and to Stacey Rodrigues and David Mider for their assistance and research. Robin Rather and David Murray were generous and tuneful hosts in Austin. Thanks also to the editors of *Women's Sports and Fitness* magazine for the patience and backing, and to Jeff Garvey for the hitched plane ride.

CONTENTS

IT'S
NOT
ABOUT
THE
BIKE

one

Before and After

I WANT TO DIE AT A HUNDRED YEARS OLD WITH an American flag on my back and the star of Texas on my helmet, after screaming down an Alpine descent on a bicycle at 75 miles per hour. I want to cross one last finish line as my stud wife and my ten children applaud, and then I want to lie down in a field of those famous French sunflowers and gracefully expire, the perfect contradiction to my once-anticipated poignant early demise.

A slow death is not for me. I don't do anything slow, not even breathe. I do everything at a fast cadence: eat fast, sleep fast. It makes me crazy when my wife, Kristin, drives our car, because she brakes at all the yellow caution lights, while I squirm impatiently in the passenger seat.

"Come on, don't be a skirt," I tell her.

"Lance," she says, "marry a man."

I've spent my life racing my bike, from the back roads of Austin, Texas to the Champs-Elysées, and I always figured if I died an untimely death, it would be because some rancher in his Dodge 4×4 ran me headfirst into a ditch. Believe me, it could happen. Cyclists fight an on-going war with guys in big trucks, and so many vehicles have hit me, so many times, in so many countries, I've lost count. I've learned how to take out my own stitches: all you need is a pair of fingernail clippers and a strong stomach.

If you saw my body underneath my racing jersey, you'd know what I'm talking about. I've got marbled scars on both arms and discolored marks up and down my legs, which I keep clean-shaven. Maybe that's why trucks are always trying to run me over; they see my sissy-boy calves and decide not to brake. But cyclists have to shave, because when the gravel gets into your skin, it's easier to clean and bandage if you have no hair.

One minute you're pedaling along a highway, and the next minute, *boom,* you're face-down in the dirt. A blast of hot air hits you, you taste the acrid, oily exhaust in the roof of your mouth, and all you can do is wave a fist at the disappearing taillights.

Cancer was like that. It was like being run off the road by a truck, and I've got the scars to prove it. There's a puckered wound in my upper chest just above my heart, which is where the catheter was implanted. A surgical line runs from the right side of my groin into my upper thigh, where they cut out my testicle. But the real prizes are two deep half-moons in my scalp, as if I was kicked twice in the head by a horse. Those are the leftovers from brain surgery.

When I was 25, I got testicular cancer and nearly died. I was given less than a 40 percent chance of surviving, and frankly, some of my doctors were just being kind when they gave me those odds. Death is not exactly cocktail-party conversation, I know, and neither is cancer, or brain surgery, or matters below the waist. But I'm not here to make polite conversation. I want to tell the truth. I'm sure you'd like to hear about how Lance Armstrong became a Great American and an Inspiration To Us All, how he won the Tour de France, the 2,290-mile road race that's considered the single most grueling sporting event on the face of the earth. You want to hear about faith and mystery, and my miraculous comeback, and how I joined towering figures like Greg LeMond and Miguel Indurain in the record book. You want to hear about my lyrical climb through the Alps and my heroic conquering of the Pyrenees, and how it *felt*. But the Tour was the least of the story.

Some of it is not easy to tell or comfortable to hear. I'm asking you now, at the outset, to put aside your ideas about heroes and miracles, because I'm not storybook material. This is not Disneyland, or Hollywood. I'll give you an example: I've read that I *flew* up the hills and mountains of France. But you don't fly up a hill. You struggle slowly and painfully up a hill, and maybe, if you work very hard, you get to the top ahead of everybody else.

Cancer is like that, too. Good, strong people get cancer, and they do all the right things to beat it, and they still die. That is the essential truth that you learn. People die. And after you learn it, all other matters seem irrelevant. They just seem small.

I don't know why I'm still alive. I can only guess. I have a tough constitution, and my profession taught me how to compete against long odds and big obstacles. I like to train hard and I like to race hard. That helped, it was a good start, but it certainly wasn't the determining factor. I can't help feeling that my survival was more a matter of blind luck.

When I was 16, I was invited to undergo testing at a place in Dallas called the Cooper Clinic, a prestigious research lab and birthplace of the aerobic exercise revolution. A doctor there measured my VO_2 max, which is a gauge of how much oxygen you can take in and use, and he says that my numbers are still the highest they've ever come across. Also, I produced less lactic acid than most people. Lactic acid is the chemical your body generates when it's winded and fatigued—it's what makes your lungs burn and your legs ache.

Basically, I can endure more physical stress than most people can, and I don't get as tired while I'm doing it. So I figure maybe that helped me live. I was lucky—I was born with an above-average capacity for breathing. But even so, I was in a desperate, sick fog much of the time.

My illness was humbling and starkly revealing, and it forced me to survey my life with an unforgiving eye. There are some shameful episodes in it: instances of meanness, unfinished tasks, weakness, and regrets. I had to ask myself, "If I live, who is it that I intend to be?" I found that I had a lot of growing to do as a man.

I won't kid you. There are two Lance Armstrongs, pre-cancer, and post. Everybody's favorite question is "How did cancer change you?" The real question is how didn't it change me? I left my house on October 2, 1996, as one person and came home another. I was a world-class athlete with a mansion on a riverbank, keys to a Porsche, and a self-made fortune in the bank. I was one of the top riders in the world and my career was moving along a perfect arc of success. I returned a different person, literally. In a way, the old me did die, and I was given a second life. Even my body is different, because during the chemotherapy I lost all the muscle I had ever built up, and when I recovered, it didn't come back in the same way.

The truth is that cancer was the best thing that ever happened to me. I don't know why I got the illness, but it did wonders for me, and I wouldn't want to walk away from it. Why would I want to change, even for a day, the most important and shaping event in my life?

People die. That truth is so disheartening that at times I can't bear to articulate it. Why should we go on, you might ask? Why don't we all just stop and lie down where we are? But there is another truth, too. People live. It's an equal and opposing truth. People live, and in the most remarkable ways. When I was sick, I saw more beauty and triumph and truth in a single day than I ever did in a bike race—but they were *human* moments, not miraculous ones. I met a guy in a fraying sweatsuit who turned out to be a brilliant surgeon. I became friends with a harassed and overscheduled nurse named LaTrice, who gave me such care that it could only be the result of the deepest sympathetic affinity. I saw children with no eyelashes or eyebrows, their hair burned away by chemo, who fought with the hearts of Indurains.

I still don't completely understand it.

All I can do is tell you what happened.

OF *course* I SHOULD HAVE KNOWN THAT SOMETHING WAS wrong with me. But athletes, especially cyclists, are in the business of denial. You deny all the aches and pains because you have to in order to finish the race. It's a sport of self-abuse. You're on your bike for the whole day, six and seven hours, in all kinds of weather and conditions, over cobblestones and gravel, in mud and wind and rain, and even hail, and you do not give in to pain.

Everything hurts. Your back hurts, your feet hurt, your hands hurt, your neck hurts, your legs hurt, and of course, your butt hurts.

So no, I didn't pay attention to the fact that I didn't feel well in 1996. When my right testicle became slightly swollen that winter, I told myself to live with it, because I assumed it was something I had done to myself on the bike, or that my system was compensating for some physiological male thing. I was riding strong, as well as I ever had, actually, and there was no reason to stop.

Cycling is a sport that rewards mature champions. It takes a physical endurance built up over years, and a head for strategy that comes only with experience. By 1996 I felt I was finally coming into my prime. That spring, I won a race called the Flèche-Wallonne, a grueling test through the Ardennes that no American had ever conquered before. I finished second in Liège-Bastogne-Liège, a classic race of 167 miles in a single punishing day. And I won the Tour Du Pont, 1,225 miles over 12 days through the Carolina mountains. I added five more second-place finishes to those results, and I was about to break into the top five in the international rankings for the first time in my career.

But cycling fans noted something odd when I won the Tour Du Pont: usually, when I won a race, I pumped my fists like pistons as I crossed the finish line. But on that day, I was too exhausted to celebrate on the bike. My eyes were bloodshot and my face was flushed.

I should have been confident and energized by my spring performances. Instead, I was just tired. My nipples were sore. If I had known better, I would have realized it was a sign of illness. It meant I had an elevated level of HCG, which is a hormone normally produced by pregnant women. Men don't have but a tiny amount of it, unless their testes are acting up.

I thought I was just run down. *Suck it up,* I said to myself, *you can't afford to be tired.* Ahead of me I still had the two most important races of the season: the Tour de France and the Olympic Games in Atlanta, and they were everything I had been training and racing for.

I dropped out of the Tour de France after just five days. I rode through a rainstorm, and developed a sore throat and bronchitis. I was coughing and had lower-back pain, and I was simply unable to get back on the bike. "I couldn't breathe," I told the press. Looking back, they were ominous words.

In Atlanta, my body gave out again. I was 6th in the time trial and 12th in the road race, respectable performances overall, but disappointing given my high expectations.

Back home in Austin, I told myself it was the flu. I was sleeping a lot, with a low-grade achy drowsy feeling. I ignored it. I wrote it off to a long hard season.

I celebrated my 25th birthday on September 18, and a couple of nights later I invited a houseful of friends over for a party before a Jimmy Buffett concert, and we rented a margarita machine. My mother Linda came over to visit from Plano, and in the midst of the party that night, I said to her, "I'm the happiest man in the world." I loved my life. I was dating a beautiful co-ed from the University of Texas named Lisa Shiels. I had just signed a new two-year contract with a prestigious French racing team, Cofidis, for $2.5 million. I had a great new house that I had spent months building, and every detail of the architectural and interior designs was exactly what I wanted. It was a Mediterranean-style home on the banks of Lake Austin, with soaring glass windows that looked out on a swimming pool and a piazza-style patio that ran down to the dock, where I had my own jet ski and powerboat moored.

Only one thing spoiled the evening: in the middle of the concert, I felt a headache coming on. It started as a dull pounding. I popped some aspirin. It didn't help. In fact, the pain got worse.

I tried ibuprofen. Now I had four tablets in me, but the headache only spread. I decided it was a case of way too many margaritas, and told myself I would never, ever drink another one. My friend and agent attorney, Bill Stapleton, bummed some migraine medication from his wife, Laura, who had a bottle in her purse. I took three. That didn't work either.

By now it was the kind of headache you see in movies, a knee-buckling, head-between-your-hands, brain-crusher.

Finally, I gave up and went home. I turned out all the lights and lay on the sofa, perfectly still. The pain never subsided, but I was so exhausted by it, and by all the tequila, that I eventually fell asleep.

When I woke up the next morning, the headache was gone. As I moved around the kitchen making coffee, I realized that my vision was a little blurry. The edges of things seemed soft. *I must be getting old,* I thought. *Maybe I need glasses.*

I had an excuse for everything.

A couple of days later, I was in my living room on the phone with Bill Stapleton when I had a bad coughing attack. I gagged, and tasted something metallic and brackish in the back of my throat. "Hang on a minute," I said. "Something's not right here." I rushed into the bathroom. I coughed into the sink.

It splattered with blood. I stared into the sink. I coughed again, and spit up another stream of red. I couldn't believe that the mass of blood and clotted matter had come from my own body.

Frightened, I went back into the living room and picked up the phone. "Bill, I have to call you back," I said. I clicked off, and immediately dialed my neighbor, Dr. Rick Parker, a good friend who was my personal physician in Austin. Rick lived just down the hill from me.

"Could you come over?" I said. "I'm coughing up blood."

While Rick was on his way, I went back into the bathroom and eyed the bloody residue in the sink. Suddenly, I turned on the faucet. I wanted to rinse it out. Sometimes I do things without knowing my own motives. I didn't want Rick to see it. I was embarrassed by it. I wanted it to go away.

Rick arrived, and checked my nose and mouth. He shined a light down my throat, and asked to see the blood. I showed him the little bit that was left in the sink. *Oh, God,* I thought, *I can't tell him how much it was, it's too disgusting.* What was left didn't look like very much.

Rick was used to hearing me complain about my sinuses and allergies. Austin has a lot of ragweed and pollen, and no matter how tortured I am, I can't take medication because of the strict doping regulations in cycling. I have to suffer through it.

"You could be bleeding from your sinuses," Rick said. "You may have cracked one."

"Great," I said. "So it's no big deal."

I was so relieved, I jumped at the first suggestion that it wasn't serious, and left it at that. Rick clicked off his flashlight, and on his way out the door he invited me to have dinner with him and his wife, Jenny, the following week.

A few nights later, I cruised down the hill to the Parkers' on a motor scooter. I have a thing for motorized toys, and the scooter was one of my favorites. But that night, I was so sore in my right testicle that it killed me to sit on the scooter. I couldn't get comfortable at the dinner table, either. I had to situate myself just right, and I didn't dare move, it was so painful.

I almost told Rick how I felt, but I was too self-conscious. It hardly seemed like something to bring up over dinner, and I had already bothered him once about the blood. *This guy is going to think I'm some kind of complainer,* I thought. I kept it to myself.

When I woke up the next morning, my testicle was horrendously swollen, almost to the size of an orange. I pulled on my clothes, got my bike from the rack in the garage, and started off on my usual training ride, but I found I couldn't even sit on the seat. I rode the whole way standing up on the pedals. When I got back home in the early afternoon, I reluctantly dialed the Parkers again.

"Rick, I've got something wrong with my testicle," I said. "It's real swollen and I had to stand up on the ride."

Rick said, sternly, "You need to get that checked out right away."

He insisted that he would get me in to see a specialist that afternoon. We hung up, and he called Dr. Jim Reeves, a prominent Austin urologist. As soon as Rick explained my symptoms, Reeves said I should come in immediately. He would hold an appointment open. Rick told me that Reeves suspected I merely had a torsion of the testicle, but that I should go in and get checked. If I ignored it, I could lose the testicle.

I showered and dressed, and grabbed my keys and got into my Porsche, and it's funny, but I can remember exactly what I wore: khaki pants and a green dress shirt. Reeves' office was in the heart of downtown, near the University of Texas campus in a plain-looking brown brick medical building.

Reeves turned out to be an older gentleman with a deep, resonating voice that sounded like it came from the bottom of a well, and a doctorly way of making everything seem routine—despite the fact that he was seriously alarmed by what he found as he examined me.

My testicle was enlarged to three times its normal size, and it was hard and painful to the touch. Reeves made some notes, and then he said, "This looks a little suspicious. Just to be safe, I'm going to send you across the street for an ultrasound."

I got my clothes back on and walked to my car. The lab was across an avenue in another institutional-looking brown brick building, and I decided to drive over. Inside was a small warren of offices and rooms filled with complicated medical equipment. I lay down on another examining table.

A female technician came in and went over me with the ultrasound equipment, a wand-like instrument that fed an image onto a screen. I figured I'd be out of there in a few minutes. Just a routine check so the doctor could be on the safe side.

An hour later, I was still on the table.

The technician seemed to be surveying every inch of me. I lay there, wordlessly, trying not to be self-conscious. Why was this taking so long? Had she found something?

Finally, she laid down the wand. Without a word, she left the room.

"Wait a minute," I said. "Hey."

I thought, *It's supposed to be a lousy formality.* After a while, she returned with a man I had seen in the office earlier. He was the chief radiologist. He picked up the wand and began to examine my parts himself. I lay there silently as he went over me for another 15 minutes. *Why is this taking so long?*

"Okay, you can get dressed and come back out," he said.

I hustled into my clothes and met him in the hallway.

"We need to take a chest X ray," he said.

I stared at him. "Why?" I said.

"Dr. Reeves asked for one," he said.

Why would they look at my chest? Nothing hurt there. I went into another examining room and took off my clothes again, and a new technician went through the X-ray process.

I was getting angry now, and scared. I dressed again, and stalked back into the main office. Down the hallway, I saw the chief radiologist.

"Hey," I said, cornering the guy. "What's going on here? This isn't normal."

"Dr. Reeves should talk to you," he said.

"No. I want to know what's going on."

"Well, I don't want to step on Dr. Reeves' toes, but it looks like perhaps he's checking you for some cancer-related activity."

I stood perfectly still.

"Oh, fuck," I said.

"You need to take the X rays back to Dr. Reeves; he's waiting for you in his office."

There was an icy feeling in the pit of my stomach, and it was growing. I took out my cell phone and dialed Rick's number.

"Rick, something's going on here, and they aren't telling me everything."

"Lance, I don't know exactly what's happening, but I'd like to go with you to see Dr. Reeves. Why don't I meet you there?"

I said, "Okay."

I waited in radiology while they prepared my X rays, and the radiologist finally came out and handed me a large brown envelope. He told me Reeves would see me in his office. I stared at the envelope. My chest was in there, I realized.

This is bad. I climbed into my car and glanced down at the envelope containing my chest X rays. Reeves' office was just 200 yards away, but it felt longer than that. It felt like two miles. Or 20.

I drove the short distance and parked. By now it was dark and well past normal office hours. If Dr. Reeves had waited for me all this time, there must be a good reason, I thought. *And the reason is that the shit is about to hit the fan.*

As I walked into Dr. Reeves' office, I noticed that the building was empty. Everyone was gone. It was dark outside.

Rick arrived, looking grim. I hunched down in a chair while Dr. Reeves opened the envelope and pulled out my X rays. An X ray is something like a photo negative: abnormalities come out white. A black image is actually good, because it means your organs are clear. Black is good. White is bad.

Dr. Reeves snapped my X rays onto a light tray in the wall.

My chest looked like a snowstorm.

"Well, this is a serious situation," Dr. Reeves said. "It looks like testicular cancer with large metastasis to the lungs."

I have cancer.

"Are you sure?" I said.

"I'm fairly sure," Dr. Reeves said.

I'm 25. Why would I have cancer?

"Shouldn't I get a second opinion?" I said.

"Of course," Dr. Reeves said. "You have every right to do that. But I should tell you I'm confident of the diagnosis. I've scheduled you for surgery tomorrow morning at 7 A.M., to remove the testicle."

I have cancer and it's in my lungs.

Dr. Reeves elaborated on his diagnosis: testicular cancer was a rare disease—only about 7,000 cases occur annually in the U.S. It tended to strike men between the ages of 18 and 25 and was considered very treatable as cancers go, thanks to advances in chemotherapy, but early diagnosis and intervention were key. Dr. Reeves was certain I had the cancer. The question was, exactly how far had it spread? He recommended that I see Dr. Dudley Youman, a renowned Austin-based oncologist. Speed was essential; every day would count. Finally, Dr. Reeves finished.

I didn't say anything.

"Why don't I leave the two of you together for a minute," Dr. Reeves said.

Alone with Rick, I laid my head down on the desk. "I just can't believe this," I said.

But I had to admit it, I was sick. The headaches, the coughing blood, the septic throat, passing out on the couch and sleeping forever. I'd had a real sick feeling, and I'd had it for a while.

"Lance, listen to me, there's been so much improvement in the treatment of cancer. It's curable. Whatever it takes, we'll get it whipped. We'll get it done."

"Okay," I said. "Okay."

Rick called Dr. Reeves back in.

"What do I have to do?" I asked. "Let's get on with it. Let's kill this stuff. Whatever it takes, let's do it."

I wanted to cure it instantly. Right away. I would have undergone surgery that night. I would have used a radiation gun on myself, if it would help. But Reeves patiently explained the procedure for the next morning: I would have to report to the hospital early for a battery of tests and blood work so the oncologist could determine the extent of the cancer, and then I would have surgery to remove my testicle.

I got up to leave. I had a lot of calls to make, and one of them was to my mother; somehow, I'd have to tell her that her only child had cancer.

I climbed into my car and made my way along the winding, tree-lined streets toward my home on the riverbank, and for the first time in my life, I drove slowly. I was in shock. *Oh, my God, I'll never be able to race again.* Not, *Oh, my God, I'll die.* Not, *Oh, my God, I'll never have a family.* Those thoughts were buried somewhere down in the confusion. But the first thing was, *Oh, my God, I'll never race again.* I picked up my car phone and called Bill Stapleton.

"Bill, I have some really bad news," I said.

"What?" he said, preoccupied.

"I'm sick. My career's over."

"What?"

"It's all over. I'm sick, I'm never going to race again, and I'm going to lose everything."

I hung up.

I drifted through the streets in first gear, without even the energy to press the gas pedal. As I puttered along, I questioned everything: my world, my profession, my self. I had left the house an indestructible 25-year-old, bulletproof. Cancer would change everything for me, I realized; it wouldn't just derail my career, it would deprive me of my entire definition of who I was. I had started with nothing. My mother was a secretary in Plano, Texas, but on my bike, I had become something. When other kids were swimming at the country club, I was biking for miles after school, because it was my chance. There were gallons of sweat all over every trophy and dollar I had ever earned, and now what would I do? Who would I be if I wasn't Lance Armstrong, world-class cyclist?

A sick person.

I pulled into the driveway of my house. Inside, the phone was ringing. I walked through the door and tossed my keys on the counter. The phone kept ringing. I picked it up. It was my friend Scott MacEachern, a representative from Nike assigned to work with me.

"Hey, Lance, what's going on?"

"Well, a lot," I said, angrily. "A lot is going on."

"What do you mean?"

"I, uh . . ."

I hadn't said it aloud yet.

"What?" Scott said.

I opened my mouth, and closed it, and opened it again. "I have cancer," I said.

I started to cry.

And then, in that moment, it occurred to me: I might lose my life, too. Not just my sport.

I could lose my life.

two

THE START LINE

YOUR PAST FORMS YOU, WHETHER YOU LIKE IT or not. Each encounter and experience has its own effect, and you're shaped the way the wind shapes a mesquite tree on a plain.

The main thing you need to know about my childhood is that I never had a real father, but I never sat around wishing for one, either. My mother was 17 when she had me, and from day one everyone told her we wouldn't amount to anything, but she believed differently, and she raised me with an unbending rule: "Make every obstacle an opportunity." And that's what we did.

I was a lot of kid, especially for one small woman. My mother's maiden name was Linda Mooneyham. She is 5-foot-3 and weighs about 105 pounds, and I don't know how somebody so tiny delivered me, because I weighed in at 9 pounds, 12 ounces. Her labor was so dif-

ficult that she lay in a fever for an entire day afterward. Her temperature was so high that the nurses wouldn't let her hold me.

I never knew my so-called father. He was a non-factor—unless
you count his absence as a factor. Just because he provided the DNA
that made me doesn't make him my father, and as far as I'm concerned, there is nothing between us, absolutely no connection. I have
no idea who he is, what he likes or dislikes. Before last year, I never
knew where he lived or worked.

I never asked. I've never had a single conversation with my mother
about him. Not once. In 28 years, she's never brought him up, and I've
never brought him up. It may seem strange, but it's true. The thing is,
I don't care, and my mother doesn't either. She says she would have
told me about him if I had asked, but frankly, it would have been like
asking a trivia question; he was that insignificant to me. I was completely loved by my mother, and I loved her back the same way, and
that felt like enough to both of us.

Since I sat down to write about my life, though, I figured I might
as well find out a few things about myself. Unfortunately, last year a
Texas newspaper traced my biological father and printed a story about
him, and this is what they reported: his name is Gunderson, and he's a
route manager for the *Dallas Morning News*. He lives in Cedar Creek
Lake, Texas, and is the father of two other children. My mother was
married to him during her pregnancy, but they split up before I was
two. He was actually quoted in the paper claiming to be a proud father,
and he said that his kids consider me their brother, but those remarks
struck me as opportunistic, and I have no interest in meeting him.

My mother was alone. Her parents were divorced, and at the time
her father, Paul Mooneyham, my grandfather, was a heavy-drinking
Vietnam vet who worked in the post office and lived in a mobile home.
Her mother, Elizabeth, struggled to support three kids. Nobody in the
family had much help to give my mother—but they tried. On the day

I was born my grandfather quit drinking, and he's been sober ever since, for 28 years, exactly as long as I've been alive. My mother's younger brother, Al, would baby-sit for me. He later joined the Army, the traditional way out for men in our family, and he made a career of it, rising all the way to the rank of lieutenant colonel. He has a lot of decorations on his chest, and he and his wife have a son named Jesse who I'm crazy about. We're proud of each other as a family.

I was wanted. My mother was so determined to have me that she hid her pregnancy by wearing baby-doll shirts so that no one would interfere or try to argue her out of it. After I was born, sometimes my mother and her sister would go grocery shopping together, and one afternoon my aunt held me while the checkout girls made cooing noises. "What a cute baby," one of them said. My mother stepped forward. "That's *my* baby," she said.

We lived in a dreary one-bedroom apartment in Oak Cliff, a suburb of Dallas, while my mother worked part-time and finished school. It was one of those neighborhoods with shirts flapping on clotheslines and a Kentucky Fried on the corner. My mother worked at the Kentucky Fried, taking orders in her pink-striped uniform, and she also punched the cash register at the Kroger's grocery store across the street. Later she got a temporary job at the post office sorting dead letters, and another one as a file clerk, and she did all of this while she was trying to study and to take care of me. She made $400 a month, and her rent was $200, and my day-care was $25 a week. But she gave me everything I needed, and a few things more. She had a way of creating small luxuries.

When I was small, she would take me to the local 7-Eleven and buy a Slurpee, and feed it to me through the straw. She would pull some up in the straw, and I would tilt my head back, and she would let the cool sweet icy drink stream into my mouth. She tried to spoil me with a 50-cent drink.

Every night she read a book to me. Even though I was just an infant, too young to understand a word, she would hold me and read. She was never too tired for that. "I can't wait until you can read to *me*," she would say. No wonder I was reciting verses by the age of two. I did everything fast. I walked at nine months.

Eventually, my mother got a job as a secretary for $12,000 a year, which allowed her to move us into a nicer apartment north of Dallas in a suburb called Richardson. She later got a job at a telecommunications company, Ericsson, and she has worked her way up the ladder. She's no longer a secretary, she's an account manager, and what's more, she got her real-estate license on the side. That right there tells you everything you need to know about her. She's sharp as a tack, and she'll outwork anybody. She also happens to look young enough to be my sister.

After Oak Cliff, the suburbs seemed like heaven to her. North Dallas stretches out practically to the Oklahoma border in an unbroken chain of suburban communities, each one exactly like the last. Tract homes and malls overrun miles of flat brown Texas landscape. But there are good schools and lots of open fields for kids to play in.

Across the street from our apartment there was a little store called the Richardson Bike Mart at one end of a strip mall. The owner was a small, well-built guy with overly bright eyes named Jim Hoyt. Jim liked to sponsor bike racers out of his store, and he was always looking to get kids started in the sport. One morning a week my mother would take me to a local shop for fresh, hot doughnuts and we would pass by the bike store. Jim knew she struggled to get by, but he noticed that she was always well turned out, and I was neat and well cared for. He took an interest in us, and gave her a deal on my first serious bike. It was a Schwinn Mag Scrambler, which I got when I was about seven. It was an ugly brown, with yellow wheels, but I loved it. Why does any kid love a bike? It's liberation and independence, your first set of wheels. A bike is freedom to roam, without rules and without adults.

There was one thing my mother gave me that I didn't particularly want—a stepfather. When I was three, my mother remarried, to a guy named Terry Armstrong. Terry was a small man with a large mustache and a habit of acting more successful than he really was. He sold food to grocery stores and he was every cliché of a traveling salesman, but he brought home a second paycheck and helped with the bills. Meanwhile, my mother was getting raises at her job, and she bought us a home in Plano, one of the more upscale suburbs.

I was a small boy when Terry legally adopted me and made my name Armstrong, and I don't remember being happy or unhappy about it, either way. All I know is that the DNA donor, Gunderson, gave up his legal rights to me. In order for the adoption to go through, Gunderson had to allow it, to agree to it. He picked up a pen and signed the papers.

Terry Armstrong was a Christian, and he came from a family who had a tendency to tell my mother how to raise me. But, for all of his proselytizing, Terry had a bad temper, and he used to whip me, for silly things. Kid things, like being messy.

Once, I left a drawer open in my bedroom, with a sock hanging out. Terry got out his old fraternity paddle. It was a thick, solid wood paddle, and frankly, in my opinion nothing like that should be used on a small boy. He turned me over and spanked me with it.

The paddle was his preferred method of discipline. If I came home late, out would come the paddle. *Whack.* If I smarted off, I got the paddle. *Whack.* It didn't hurt just physically, but also emotionally. So I didn't like Terry Armstrong. I thought he was an angry testosterone geek, and as a result, my early impression of organized religion was that it was for hypocrites.

Athletes don't have much use for poking around in their childhoods, because introspection doesn't get you anywhere in a race. You don't want to think about your adolescent resentments when you're trying to make a 6,500-foot climb with a cadre of Italians and Spaniards on your wheel. You need a dumb focus. But that said, it's all stoked down in there, fuel for the fire. "Make every negative into a positive," as my mother says. Nothing goes to waste, you put it all to use, the old wounds and long-ago slights become the stuff of competitive energy. But back then I was just a kid with about four chips on his shoulder, thinking, *Maybe if I ride my bike on this road long enough it will take me out of here.*

Plano had its effect on me, too. It was the quintessential American suburb, with strip malls, perfect grid streets, and faux-antebellum country clubs in between empty brown wasted fields. It was populated by guys in golf shirts and Sansabelt pants, and women in bright fake gold jewelry, and alienated teenagers. Nothing there was old, nothing real. To me, there was something soul-deadened about the place, which may be why it had one of the worst heroin problems in the country, as well as an unusually large number of teen suicides. It's home to Plano East High School, one of the largest and most football-crazed high schools in the state, a modern structure that looks more like a government agency, with a set of doors the size of loading docks. That's where I went to school.

In Plano, Texas, if you weren't a football player you didn't exist, and if you weren't upper middle class, you might as well not exist either. My mother was a secretary, so I tried to play football. But I had no coordination. When it came to anything that involved moving from side to side, or hand-eye coordination—when it came to anything involving a ball, in fact—I was no good.

I was determined to find something I could succeed at. When I was in fifth grade, my elementary school held a distance-running race. I told my mother the night before the race, "I'm going to be a champ." She just looked at me, and then she went into her things and dug out a 1972 silver dollar. "This is a good-luck coin," she said. "Now remember, all you have to do is beat that clock." I won the race.

A few months later, I joined the local swim club. At first it was another way to seek acceptance with the other kids in the suburbs, who all swam laps at Los Rios Country Club, where their parents were members. On the first day of swim practice, I was so inept that I was put with the seven-year-olds. I looked around, and saw the younger sister of one of my friends. It was embarrassing. I went from not being any good at football to not being any good at *swimming*.

But I tried. If I had to swim with the little kids to learn technique, then that's what I was willing to do. My mother gets emotional to this day when she remembers how I leaped headfirst into the water and flailed up and down the length of the pool, as if I was trying to splash all the water out of it. "You tried so *hard*," she says. I didn't swim in the worst group for long.

Swimming is a demanding sport for a 12-year-old, and the City of Plano Swim Club was particularly intense. I swam for a man named Chris MacCurdy, who remains one of the best coaches I ever worked with. Within a year, Chris transformed me; I was fourth in the state in the 1,500-meter freestyle. He trained our team seriously: we had workouts every morning from 5:30 to 7. Once I got a little older I began to ride my bike to practice, ten miles through the semi-dark early-morning streets. I would swim 4,000 meters of laps before school and go back for another two-hour workout in the afternoon—another 6,000 meters. That was six miles a day in the water, plus a 20-mile bike ride. My mother let me do it for two reasons: she didn't have the option of driving me herself because she worked, and she knew that I needed to channel my temperament.

One afternoon when I was about 13 and hanging around the Richardson Bike Mart, I saw a flyer for a competition called IronKids.

It was a junior triathlon, an event that combined biking, swimming, and running. I had never heard of a triathlon before—but it was all of the things I was good at, so I signed up. My mother took me to a shop and bought me a triathlon outfit, which basically consisted of cross-training shorts and a shirt made out of a hybrid fast-drying material, so I could wear it through each phase of the event, without changing. We got my first racing bike then, too. It was a Mercier, a slim, elegant road bike.

I won, and I won by a lot, without even training for it. Not long afterward, there was another triathlon, in Houston. I won that, too. When I came back from Houston, I was full of self-confidence. I was a top junior at swimming, but I had never been the absolute best at it. I was better at triathlons than any kid in Plano, and any kid in the whole state, for that matter. I liked the feeling.

What makes a great endurance athlete is the ability to absorb potential embarrassment, and to suffer without complaint. I was discovering that if it was a matter of gritting my teeth, not caring how it looked, and outlasting everybody else, I won. It didn't seem to matter what the sport was—in a straight-ahead, long-distance race, I could beat anybody.

If it was a suffer-fest, I was good at it.

I COULD HAVE DEALT WITH TERRY ARMSTRONG'S PADdle. But there was something else I couldn't deal with.

When I was 14, my mother went into the hospital to have a hysterectomy. It's a very tough operation for any woman, physically and emotionally, and my mother was still very young when it happened. I was entered in a swim meet in San Antonio, so I had to leave while she was still recuperating, and Terry decided to chaperone me. I didn't want him there; I didn't like it when he tried to play Little League Dad, and I thought he should be at the hospital. But he insisted.

As we sat in the airport waiting for our flight, I gazed at Terry and thought, *Why are you here?* As I watched him, he began to write notes on a pad. He would write, then ball up the paper and throw it into the garbage can and start again. I thought it was peculiar. After a while Terry got up to go to the bathroom. I went over to the garbage can, retrieved the wadded papers, and stuffed them into my bag.

Later, when I was alone, I took them out and unfolded them. They were to another woman. I read them, one by one. He was writing to another woman while my mother was in the hospital having a hysterectomy.

I flew back to Dallas with the crumpled pages in the bottom of my bag. When I got home, I went to my room and pulled my copy of *The Guinness Book of World Records* off the shelf. I got a pair of scissors, and hollowed out the center of the book. I crammed the pages into the hollow and stuck the book back on the shelf. I wanted to keep the pages, and I'm not quite sure why. For insurance, maybe; a little ammunition, in case I ever needed it. In case Terry decided to use the paddle again.

If I hadn't liked Terry before, from then on, I felt nothing for him. I didn't respect him, and I began to challenge his authority.

Let me sum up my turbulent youth. When I was a boy, I invented a game called fireball, which entailed soaking a tennis ball in kerosene, lighting it on fire, and playing catch with it wearing a pair of garden gloves.

I'd fill a plastic dish-tub full of gasoline, and then I'd empty a can of tennis balls into the tub and let them float there. I'd fish one out and hold a match to it, and my best friend Steve Lewis and I would throw the blazing ball back and forth until our gloves smoked. Imagine it, two boys standing in a field in a hot Texas breeze, pitching flames at each other. Sometimes the gardening gloves would catch on fire, and we'd flap them against our jeans, until embers flew into the air around our heads, like fireflies.

Once, I accidentally threw the ball up onto the roof. Some shingles caught fire, and I had to scramble up there and stamp out the fire before it burned down the whole house and then started on the neighbors' place. Then there was the time a tennis ball landed squarely in the middle of the tray full of gas, and the whole works exploded. It went *up,* a wall of flame and a swirling tower of black smoke. I panicked and kicked over the tub, trying to put the fire out. Instead, the tub started melting down into the ground, like something out of *The China Syndrome.*

A lot of my behavior had to do with knowing that my mother wasn't happy; I couldn't understand why she would stay with Terry when they seemed so miserable. But being with him probably seemed better to her than raising a son on her own and living on one paycheck.

A few months after the trip to San Antonio, the marriage finally fell apart. One evening I was going to be late for dinner, so I called my mother. She said, "Son, you need to come home."

"What's wrong?" I said.

"I need to talk to you."

I got on my bike and rode home, and when I got there, she was sitting in the living room.

"I told Terry to leave," she said. "I'm going to file for divorce."

I was beyond relieved, and I didn't bother to hide it. In fact, I was downright joyful. "This is great," I said, beaming.

"But, son," she said, "I don't want you to give me any problems. I can't handle that right now. Please, just don't give me any problems."

"All right," I said. "I promise."

I waited a few weeks to say anything more about it. But then one day when we were sitting around in the kitchen, out of the blue, I said to my mother, "That guy was no good." I didn't tell her about the letters—she was unhappy enough. But years later, when she was cleaning, she found them. She wasn't surprised.

For a while, Terry tried to stay in touch with me by sending birthday cards and things like that. He would send an envelope with a hundred one-dollar bills in it. I'd take it to my mother and say, "Would you please send this back to him? I don't want it." Finally, I wrote him a letter telling him that if I could, I would change my name. I didn't feel I had a relationship with him, or with his family.

After the breakup, my mother and I grew much closer. I think she had been unhappy for a while, and when people are unhappy, they're not themselves. She changed once she got divorced. She was more relaxed, as if she had been under some pressure and now it was gone. Of course, she was under another kind of pressure as a single woman again, trying to support both of us, but she had been through that before. She was single for the next five years.

I tried to be dependable. I'd climb on our roof to put up the Christmas lights for her—and if I mooned the cars on the avenue, well, that was a small, victimless crime. When she got home from work, we would sit down to dinner together, and turn off the TV, and we'd talk. She taught me to eat by candlelight, and insisted on decent manners. She would fix a taco salad or a bowl of Hamburger Helper, light the candles, and tell me about her day. Sometimes she would talk about how frustrated she was at work, where she felt she was underestimated because she was a secretary.

"Why don't you quit?" I asked.

"Son, you never quit," she said. "I'll get through it."

Sometimes she would come home and I could see she'd had a really bad day. I'd be playing something loud on the stereo, like Guns 'N

Roses, but I'd take one look at her and turn the heavy stuff off, and put something else on. "Mom, this is for you," I'd say. And I'd play Kenny G for her—which believe me was a sacrifice.

I tried to give her emotional support, because she did so many small things for me. Little things. Every Saturday, she would wash and iron five shirts, so that I had a freshly pressed shirt for each school day of the week. She knew how hard I trained and how hungry I got in the afternoons, so she would leave a pot of homemade spaghetti sauce in the refrigerator, for a snack. She taught me to boil my own pasta and how to throw a strand against the wall to make sure it was done.

I was beginning to earn my own money. When I was 15, I entered the 1987 President's Triathlon in Lake Lavon, against a field of experienced older athletes. I finished 32nd, shocking the other competitors and spectators, who couldn't believe a 15-year-old had held up over the course. I got some press coverage for that race, and I told a reporter, "I think in a few years I'll be right near the top, and within ten years I'll be the best." My friends, guys like Steve Lewis, thought I was hilariously cocky. (The next year, I finished fifth.)

Triathlons paid good money. All of a sudden I had a wallet full of first-place checks, and I started entering triathlons wherever I could find them. Most of the senior ones had age restrictions—you had to be 16 or older to enter—so I would doctor my birth date on the entry form to meet the requirements. I didn't win in the pros, but I would place in the top five. The other competitors started calling me "Junior."

But if it sounds like it came easy, it didn't. In one of the first pro triathlons I entered, I made the mistake of eating badly beforehand— I downed a couple of cinnamon rolls and two Cokes—and I paid for it by bonking, meaning I ran completely out of energy. I had an empty tank. I was first out of the water, and first off the bike. But in the middle of the run, I nearly collapsed. My mother was waiting at the finish, accustomed to seeing me come in among the leaders, and she couldn't understand what was taking me so long. Finally, she walked out on the course and found me, struggling along.

"Come on, son, you can do it," she said.

"I'm totally gone," I said. "I bonked."

"All right," she said. "But you can't quit, either. Even if you have to walk to the finish line."

I walked to the finish line.

I began to make a name in local bike races, too. On Tuesday nights there was a series of criteriums—multi-lap road races—held on an old loop around those empty Richardson fields. The Tuesday-night "crits" were hotly contested among serious local club riders, and they drew a large crowd. I rode for Hoyt, who sponsored a club team out of the Richardson Bike Mart, and my mother got me a toolbox to hold all of my bike stuff. She says she can still remember me pedaling around the loop, powering past other kids, lapping the field. She couldn't believe how strong I was. I didn't care if it was just a $100 cash prize, I would tear the legs off the other riders to get at it.

There are degrees of competitive cycling, and they are rated by category, with Category 1 being the highest level, Category 4 the lowest. I started out in the "Cat 4" races at the Tuesday-night crits, but I was anxious to move up. In order to do so you had to have results, win a certain number of races. But I was too impatient for that, so I convinced the organizers to let me ride in the Cat 3 race with the older and more experienced group. The organizers told me, "Okay, but whatever you do, don't win." If I drew too much attention to myself, there might be a big stink about how they had let me skip the requirements.

I won. I couldn't help it. I dusted the other riders. Afterward there was some discussion about what to do with me, and one option was suspending me. Instead, they upgraded me. There were three or four men around there who were Cat 1 riders, local heroes, and they all rode for the Richardson Bike Mart, so I began training with them, a 16-year-old riding with guys in their late 20s.

By now I was the national rookie of the year in sprint triathlons, and my mother and I realized that I had a future as an athlete. I was making about $20,000 a year, and I began keeping a Rolodex full of business contacts. I needed sponsors and supporters who were willing to front my airfare and my expenses to various races. My mother told me, "Look, Lance, if you're going to get anywhere, you're going to have to do it yourself, because no one is going to do it for you."

My mother had become my best friend and most loyal ally. She was my organizer and my motivator, a dynamo. "If you can't give 110 percent, you won't make it," she would tell me.

She brought an organizational flair to my training. "Look, I don't know what you need," she'd say. "But I recommend that you sit down and do a mental check of everything, because you don't want to get there and not have it." I was proud of her, and we were very much alike; we understood each other perfectly, and when we were together we didn't have to say much. We just knew. She always found a way to get me the latest bike I wanted, or the accessories that went with it. In fact, she still has all of my discarded gears and pedals, because they were so expensive she couldn't bear to get rid of them.

We traveled all over together, entering me in 10K runs and triathlons. We even began to think that I could be an Olympian. I still carried the silver-dollar good-luck piece, and now she gave me a key chain that said "1988" on it—the year of the next summer Olympics.

Every day after school I'd run six miles, and then get on my bike and ride into the evening. I learned to love Texas on those rides. The countryside was beautiful, in a desolate kind of way. You could ride out on the back roads through vast ranchland and cotton fields with nothing in the distance but water towers, grain elevators, and dilapidated sheds. The grass was chewed to nubs by livestock and the dirt looked like what's left in the bottom of an old cup of coffee. Sometimes I'd find rolling fields of wildflowers, and solitary mesquite trees blown into strange shapes. But other times the countryside was just flat yellowish-brown prairie, with the occasional gas station, everything fields, fields of brown grass, fields of cotton, just flat and awful, and windy. Dallas is the third-windiest city in the country. But it was good for me. Resistance.

One afternoon I got run off the road by a truck. By then, I had discovered my middle finger, and I flashed it at the driver. He pulled over, and threw a gas can at me, and came after me. I ran, leaving my beautiful Mercier bike by the side of the road. The guy stomped on it, damaging it.

Before he drove off I got his license number, and my mom took the guy to court, and won. In the meantime, she got me a new bike with her insurance, a Raleigh with racing wheels.

Back then I didn't have an odometer on my bike, so if I wanted to know how long a training ride was, my mother would have to drive it. If I told her I needed to measure the ride, she got in the car, even if it was late. Now, a 30-odd-mile training ride is nothing for me, but for a woman who just got off work it's long enough to be a pain to drive. She didn't complain.

My mother and I became very open with each other. She trusted me, totally. I did whatever I wanted, and the interesting thing is that no matter what I did, I always told her about it. I never lied to her. If I wanted to go out, nobody stopped me. While most kids were sneaking out of their houses at night, I'd go out through the front door.

I probably had too much rope. I was a hyper kid, and I could have done some harm to myself. There were a lot of wide boulevards and fields in Plano, an invitation to trouble for a teenager on a bike or behind the wheel of a car. I'd weave up and down the avenues on my bike, dodging cars and racing the stoplights, going as far as downtown Dallas. I used to like to ride in traffic, for the challenge.

My brand-new Raleigh was top-of-the-line and beautiful, but I owned it only a short time before I wrecked it and almost got myself killed. It happened one afternoon when I was running stoplights. I was spinning through them one after the other, trying to beat the timers. I got five of them. Then I came to a giant intersection of two six-lanes, and the light turned yellow.

I kept going anyway—which I did all the time. Still do.

I got across three lanes before the light turned red. As I raced across the fourth lane, I saw a lady in a Ford Bronco out of the corner of my eye. She didn't see me. She accelerated—and smashed right into me.

I went flying, headfirst across the intersection. No helmet. Landed on my head, and just kind of rolled to a stop at the curb.

I was alone. I had no ID, nothing on me. I tried to get up. But then there were people crowding around me, and somebody said, "No, no, don't move!" I lay back down and waited for the ambulance while the lady who'd hit me had hysterics. The ambulance arrived and took me to the hospital, where I was conscious enough to recite my phone number, and the hospital people called my mother, who got pretty hysterical, too.

I had a concussion, and I took a bunch of stitches in my head, and a few more in my foot, which was gashed wide open. The car had broadsided me, so my knee was sprained and torn up, and it had to be put in a heavy brace. As for the bike, it was completely mangled.

I explained to the doctor who treated me that I was in training for a triathlon to be held six days later at Lake Dallas in Louisville. The doctor said, "Absolutely no way. You can't do anything for three weeks. Don't run, don't walk."

I left the hospital a day later, limping and sore and thinking I was out of action. But after a couple of days of sitting around, I got bored. I went out to play golf at a little local course, even though I still had the leg brace on. It felt good to be out and be moving around. I took the leg brace off. I thought, *Well, this isn't so bad.*

By the fourth day, I didn't see what the big deal was. I felt pretty good. I signed up for the triathlon, and that night I told my mother, "I'm doing that thing. I'm racing."

She just said, "Okay. Great."

I called a friend and said, "I gotta borrow your bike." Then I went into my bathroom and cut the stitches out of my foot. I was already good with the nail clippers. I left the ones in my head, since I'd be wearing a swim cap. Then I cut holes in my running shoe and my bike shoe so the gash in my foot wouldn't rub.

Early the next morning, I was at the starting line with the rest of the competitors. I was first out of the water. I was first off the bike. I got caught by a couple of guys on the 10K run, and took third. The next day, there was a big article in the paper about how I'd been hit by a car and still finished third. A week later, my mom and I got a letter from the doctor. "I can't believe it," he wrote.

NOTHING SEEMED TO SLOW ME DOWN. I HAVE A LOVE of acceleration in any form, and as a teenager I developed a fascination with high-performance cars. The first thing I did with the prize money from my triathlon career was buy a little used red Fiat, which I would race around Plano—without a driver's license.

One afternoon when I was in 11th grade, I pulled off a serious piece of driving that my old friends still marvel at. I was cruising down a two-lane road with some classmates when we approached two cars moving slowly.

Impatiently, I hit the gas.

I drove my little Fiat right between the two cars. I shot the gap, and you could have stuck your finger out of the window and into the open mouths of the other drivers.

I took the car out at night, which was illegal unless an adult was with me. One Christmas season, I got a part-time job working at Toys "Я" Us, helping carry stuff out to customers' cars. Steve Lewis got a job at Target, and we both had night shifts, so our parents let us take the cars to work. Bad decision. Steve and I would drag-race home, doing 80 or 90 through the streets.

Steve had a Pontiac Trans Am, and I upgraded to a Camaro IROC Z28, a monster of a car. I was in a cheesy disco phase, and I wanted that car more than anything. Jim Hoyt helped me buy it by signing the loan, and I made all the monthly payments and carried the insurance. It was a fast, fast car, and some nights, we'd go down to Forest Lane, which was a drag-strip area, and get it up to 115 or 120 mph, down a 45-mph road.

I had two sets of friends, a circle of popular high-school kids who I would carouse with, and then my athlete friends, the bike racers and runners and triathletes, some of them grown men. There was social pressure at Plano East, but my mother and I couldn't begin to keep up with the Joneses, so we didn't even try. While other kids drove hot cars that their parents had given them, I drove the one I had bought with my own money.

Still, I felt shunned at times. I was the guy who did weird sports and who didn't wear the right labels. Some of my more social friends would say things like, "If I were you, I'd be embarrassed to wear those Lycra shorts." I shrugged. There was an unwritten dress code; the so-cially acceptable people all wore uniforms with Polo labels on them. They might not have known it, but that's what they were: uniforms. Same pants, same boots, same belts, same wallets, same caps. It was total conformity, and everything I was against.

IN THE FALL OF MY SENIOR YEAR IN HIGH SCHOOL I entered an important time trial in Moriarty, New Mexico, a big race for young riders, on a course where it was easy to ride a fast time. It was a flat 12 miles with very little wind, along a stretch of highway. A lot of big trucks passed through, and they would belt you with a hot blast of air that pushed you along. Young riders went there to set records and get noticed.

It was September but still hot when we left Texas, so I packed light. On the morning of my ride I got up at 6 and headed out the door into a blast of early-morning mountain air. All I had on was a pair of bike shorts and a short-sleeved racing jersey. I got five minutes down the road, and thought, *I can't handle this.* It was frigid.

I turned around and went back to the room. I said, "Mom, it's so cold out there I can't ride. I need a jacket or something." We looked through our luggage, and I didn't have a single piece of warm clothing. I hadn't brought anything. I was totally unprepared. It was the act of a complete amateur.

My mom said, "Well, I have a little windbreaker that I brought," and she pulled out this tiny pink jacket. I've told you how small and delicate she is. It looked like something a doll would wear.

"I'll take it," I said. It was that cold.

I went back outside. The sleeves came up to my elbows, and it was tight all over, but I wore it all through my warmup, a 45-minute ride. I still had it on when I got to the starting area. Staying warm is critical for a time trial, because when they say "go," you've got to be completely ready to go, *boom,* all-out for 12 miles. But I was still cold.

Desperate, I said, "Mom, get in the car, and turn on the heat as hot and high as it'll go."

She started the car and let it run, and put the heat on full blast. I got in and huddled in front of the heating vents. I said, "Just tell me when it's time to go." That was my warmup.

Finally, it was my turn. I got out of the car and right onto the bike. I went to the start line and took off. I smashed the course record by 45 seconds.

The things that were important to people in Plano were becoming less and less important to me. School and socializing were second to me now; developing into a world-class athlete was first. My life's ambition wasn't to own a tract home near a strip mall. I had a fast car and money in my wallet, but that was because I was winning races—in sports none of my classmates understood or cared about.

I took longer and longer training rides by myself. Sometimes a bunch of us would go camping or waterskiing, and afterward, instead of riding home in a car with everyone else, I'd cycle all the way back alone. Once, after a camping trip in Texoma with some buddies, I rode 60 miles home.

Not even the teachers at school seemed to understand what I was after. During the second semester of my senior year, I was invited by the U.S. Cycling Federation to go to Colorado Springs to train with the junior U.S. national team, and to travel to Moscow for my first big international bike race, the 1990 Junior World Championships. Word had gotten around after my performance in New Mexico.

But the administrators at Plano East objected. They had a strict policy: no unexcused absences. You'd think a trip to Moscow would be worth extra credits, and you'd think a school would be proud to have an Olympic prospect in its graduation rolls. But they didn't care.

I went to Colorado Springs anyway, and then to Moscow. At the Junior Worlds, I had no idea what I was doing, I was all raw energy with no concept of pacing or tactics. But I led for several laps anyway, before I faded, out of gas from attacking too early. Still, the U.S. federation officials were impressed, and the Russian coach told everybody I was the best young cyclist he had seen in years.

I was gone for six weeks. When I got back in March, my grades were all zeroes because of the missed attendance. A team of six administrators met with my mother and me, and told us that unless I made up all of the work in every subject over just a few weeks, I wouldn't graduate with my class. My mother and I were stunned.

"But there's no way I can do that," I told them.

The suits just looked at me.

"You're not a quitter, are you?" one of them said.

I stared back at them. I knew damn well that if I played football and wore Polo shirts and had parents who belonged to Los Rios Country Club, things would be different.

"This meeting is over," I said.

We got up and walked out. We had already paid for the graduation announcements, the cap and gown, and the senior prom. My mother said, "You stay in school for the rest of the day, and by the time you get home, I'll have this worked out."

She went back to her office and called every private school in the Dallas phone book. She would ask a private school to accept me, and then confess that she couldn't pay for the tuition, so could they take me for free? She dialed schools all over the area and explained our dilemma. "He's not a bad kid," she'd plead. "He doesn't do drugs. I promise you, he's going places."

By the end of the day, she'd found a private academy, Bending Oaks, that was willing to accept me if I took a couple of make-up courses. We transferred all of my credits from Plano East, and I got my degree on time. At the graduation ceremony, all of my classmates had maroon tassels on their caps, while mine was Plano East gold, but I wasn't a bit embarrassed.

I decided to go to my senior prom at Plano East anyway. We'd already paid for it, so I wasn't about to miss it. I bought a corsage for my date, rented a tuxedo, and booked a limousine. That night, as I was getting dressed in my tux and bow tie, I had an idea. My mother had never been in a limo.

I wanted her to experience that ride. How do you articulate all that you feel for and owe to a parent? My mother had given me more than any teacher or father figure ever had, and she had done it over some long hard years, years that must have looked as empty to her at times as those brown Texas fields. When it came to never quitting, to not caring how it looked, to gritting your teeth and pushing to the finish, I could only hope to have the stamina and fortitude of my mother, a single woman with a young son and a small salary—and there was no reward for her at the end of the day, either, no trophy or first-place check. For her, there was just the knowledge that honest effort was a transforming experience, and that her love was redemptive. Every time she said, "Make an obstacle an opportunity, make a negative a positive," she was talking about me, I realized; about her decision to have me and the way she had raised me.

"Get your prom dress on," I told her.

She owned a beautiful sundress that she liked to call her "prom dress," so she put it on and got in the car with my date and me, and together we rode around town for more than an hour, laughing and toasting my graduation, until it was time to drop us off at the dance.

My mother was happy again, and settling into a new relationship. When I was 17, she met a man named John Walling, a good guy who she eventually married. I liked him, and we became friends, and I would be sorry when they split up in 1998.

It's funny. People are always saying to me, "Hey, I ran into your father." I have to stop and think, *Exactly who do they mean?* It could be any of three people, and frankly, my birth father I don't know from a bank teller, and I have nothing to say to Terry. Occasionally, some of the Armstrongs try to get in touch with me, as if we're family. But we aren't related, and I wish they would respect my feelings on the subject. My family are the Mooneyhams. As for Armstrong, it's as if I made up my name, that's how I feel about it.

I'm sure the Armstrongs would give you 50,000 different reasons why I needed a father, and what great jobs they did. But I disagree. My mother gave me everything. All I felt for them was a kind of coldness, and a lack of trust.

FOR A FEW MONTHS AFTER GRADUATION, I HUNG around Plano. Most of my Plano East classmates went on to the state-university system; my buddy Steve, for instance, got his degree from North Texas State in 1993. (Not long ago, Plano East held its 10th reunion. I wasn't invited.)

I was getting tired of living in Plano. I was competing in bike races all over the country for a domestic trade team sponsored by Subaru–Montgomery, but I knew the real racing scene was in Europe, and I felt I should be there. Also, I had too much resentment for the place after what had happened before my graduation.

I was in limbo. By now I was regularly beating the adult men I competed against, whether in a triathlon, or a 10K run, or a Tuesday-night crit at the Plano loop. To pass the time, I still hung around the Richardson Bike Mart, owned by Jim Hoyt.

Jim had been an avid rider as a young man, but then he got shipped off to Vietnam when he was 19, and served two years in the infantry, the toughest kind of duty. When he came home, all he wanted to do was ride a bike again. He started out as a distributor for Schwinn, and then he opened his own store with his wife, Rhonda. For years Jim and Rhonda have cultivated young riders in the Dallas area by fronting them bikes and equipment, and by paying them stipends. Jim believed in performance incentives. We would compete for cash and free stuff he'd put up, and we raced that much harder because of it. All through my senior year in high school, I earned $500 a month riding for Jim Hoyt.

Jim had a small office in the back of his store where we'd sit around and talk. I didn't pay much attention to school principals, or stepfathers, but sometimes I liked to talk to him. "I work my butt off, but I love who I am," he'd say. "If you judge everybody by money, you got a lot to learn as you move through this life, 'cause I got some friends who own their own companies, and I got some friends who mow yards." But Jim was tough too, and you didn't fool with him. I had a healthy respect for his temper.

One night at the Tuesday crits, I got into a sprint duel with another rider, an older man I wasn't real fond of. As we came down the final stretch, our bikes made contact. We crossed the finish line shoving each other, and we were throwing punches before our bikes came to a stop. Then we were on each other, in the dirt. Jim and some others finally pried us apart, and everybody laughed at me because I wanted to keep duking it out. But Jim got mad at me, and wasn't going to allow that kind of thing. He walked over and picked up my bike, and wheeled it away. I was sorry to see it go.

It was a Schwinn Paramount, a great bike that I had ridden in Moscow at the World Championships, and I wanted to use it again in a stage race the following week. A little later, I went over to Jim's house. He came out into the front yard.

"Can I have my bike back?" I said.

"Nope," he said. "You want to talk to me, you come to my office tomorrow."

I backed away from him. He was irate, to the point that I was afraid he might take a swing at me. And there was something else he wasn't too happy about: he knew I had a habit of speeding in the Camaro.

A few days later, he took the car back, too. I was beside myself. I had made all the payments on that car, about $5,000 worth. On the other hand, some of that money had come from the stipend he paid me to ride for his team. But I wasn't thinking clearly, I was too mad. When you're 17 and a man takes a Camaro IROC Z away from you, he's on your hit list. So I never did go see Jim. I was too angry, and too afraid of him.

It was years before we spoke again.

Instead, I split town. After my visit to Colorado Springs and Moscow, I was named to the U.S. national cycling team, and I got a call from Chris Carmichael, the team's newly named director. Chris had heard about my reputation; I was super strong, but I didn't understand a lot about the tactics of racing. Chris told me he wanted to develop a whole new group of young American cyclists; the sport was stagnant in the U.S. and he was seeking fresh kids to rejuvenate it. He named some other young cyclists who showed potential, guys like Bobby Julich and George Hincapie, and said he wanted me to be one of them. How would I like to go to Europe?

It was time to get out of the house.

three

I Don't Check My Mother at the Door

THE LIFE OF A ROAD CYCLIST MEANS HAVING your feet clamped to the bike pedals churning at 20 to 40 miles per hour, for hours and hours and days on end across whole continents. It means gulping water and wolfing candy bars in the saddle because you lose 10 to 12 liters of fluid and burn 6,000 calories a day at such a pace, and you don't stop for anything, not even to piss, or to put on a raincoat. Nothing interrupts the high-speed chess match that goes on in the tight pack of cyclists called the *peloton* as you hiss through the rain and labor up cold mountainsides, swerving over rain-slick pavement and jouncing over cobblestones, knowing that a single wrong move by a nervous rider who grabs his brakes too hard or yanks too sharply on his handlebars can turn you and your bike into a heap of twisted metal and scraped flesh.

I had no idea what I was getting into. When I left home at 18, my idea of a race was to leap on and start pedaling. I was called "brash" in my early days, and the tag has followed me ever since, maybe deservedly. I was very young and I had a lot to learn, and I said and did some things that maybe I shouldn't have, but I wasn't trying to be a jerk. I was just Texan. The *"Toro de Texas,"* the Spanish press named me.

In my first big international race, I did everything my coach told me *not* to do. It was at the 1990 amateur World Championships in Utsunomiya, Japan, a 115-mile road race over a tough course with a long, hard climb. To make matters more difficult, it happened to be a sweltering day with temperatures in the 90s. I was competing as a member of the U.S. national team under Chris Carmichael, a sandy-haired, freckled young coach who I didn't know very well yet—and didn't listen to.

Chris gave me strict instructions: I was to hang back in the pack for much of the race and look for his signal before making any kind of move. It was too hot and the course too arduous to try to race in front, into the headwind. The smart thing to do was to draft and conserve my energy.

"I want you to wait," Chris said. "I don't want to see you near the front, catching any wind."

I nodded, and moved to the start area. On the first lap, I did what he told me to and rode near the back. But then I couldn't help myself; I wanted to test my legs. I began to move up. On the second lap, I took the lead, and when I came by the checkpoint, I was all by myself, 45 seconds up on the field. I streaked past Chris. As I went by, I glanced over at him. He had his arms spread wide, as if to say, "What are you doing?"

I grinned at him and gave him the Texas Longhorn sign: I waved, my pinky and forefinger extended in the air. *Hook 'em, horns.*

Chris started yelling to the U.S. staff, "What is he *doing?*"

What was I doing? I was just going. It was a move that would become known as classic early Armstrong: a contrary and spectacularly ill-advised attack. I proceeded to go solo for the next three laps, and built a lead of about a minute and a half. I was feeling pretty good about myself, when the heat started to get to me. Next thing I knew, 30 guys came up and joined me. With half the race still to go, I was already suffering. I tried to keep riding at the front, but I didn't have enough left. Sapped by the heat and the climbs, I finished 11th.

Still, it was the best American finish in the history of the race, and by the time it ended, Chris was more pleased than angry. Afterward, we went to the hotel bar and drank a beer together and talked. I wasn't sure how I felt about Chris. When I first came out of Plano he had split the U.S. national team into two groups, and placed me with the "B" team, and I hadn't quite forgiven him for the slight. I would learn, however, that his easygoing manner came with a brotherly loyalty and a vast amount of cycling wisdom; he was a former Olympian, and had competed with Greg LeMond as a young cyclist.

We sipped Kirin and went over the events of the day, laughing about them. Then suddenly Chris turned serious. He congratulated me for the 11th-place finish, and said he liked what he saw. "You weren't afraid to fail," he said. "You weren't out there thinking, 'What if I get caught?' " I absorbed the praise happily.

But then he added, "Of course, if you had known what you were doing and conserved your energy, you'd have been in the medals."

Here I had done better than any American ever before, and Chris was suggesting it wasn't good enough. In fact, in his subtle way, he was telling me that I had blown it. He kept talking. "I'm serious. You can do a lot better," he said. "I'm convinced you're going to be a world champion. But there's a lot of work to do."

Chris pointed out that the top riders, the Marco Pantanis, the Miguel Indurains, were all as strong as or stronger than I was. "So is everybody you're racing at this level," he said. What would separate me would be my tactics.

I had to learn how to race, and the only place to do it was on the bike. That first year, I must have spent 200 days overseas, riding around Europe, because the true test was on the road, where there was no hiding in a 160-mile race. In the last part, you either had it or you didn't.

At home, I settled in Austin, in the Texas hill country where stony, dark-green banks surround the town lake that's fed by the wide, uneasy waters of the Colorado River. In Austin, nobody seemed to care what I wore, or whether I "belonged" or not. In fact, I couldn't find two people dressed alike, and some of the wealthiest people in town looked like vagrants. It was a town that seemed to be made for the young, with an ever-evolving selection of bars and music clubs on 6th Street, and hole-in-the-wall Tex-Mex joints where I could eat chili peppers for sport.

It was also a great town for training, with endless bike trails and back roads to explore for miles around. I rented a small bungalow near the University of Texas campus, which was fitting since I was a student, not in the classroom, of course, but on the bike.

Cycling is an intricate, highly politicized sport, and it's far more of a team sport than the spectator realizes, as I was discovering. It has a language all its own, pieced together from a sampling of European words and phrases, and a peculiar ethic as well. On any team, each rider has a job, and is responsible for a specific part of the race. The slower riders are called *domestiques*—servants—because they do the less glamorous work of "pulling" up hills ("pulling" is cycling lingo for blocking the wind for the other riders) and protecting their team leader through the various perils of a stage race. The team leader is the principal cyclist, the rider most capable of sprinting to a finish with 150 miles in his legs. I was starting as a domestique, but I would gradually be groomed for the role of team leader.

I learned about the peloton—the massive pack of riders that makes up the main body of the race. To the spectator it seems like a radiant blur, humming as it goes by, but that colorful blur is rife with contact, the clashing of handlebars, elbows, and knees, and it's full of international intrigues and deals. The speed of the peloton varies. Sometimes it moves at 20 miles an hour, the riders pedaling slow and chatting. Other times, the group is spanned out across the road and we're going 40 miles an hour. Within the peloton, there are constant negotiations between competing riders: pull me today, and I'll pull you tomorrow. Give an inch, make a friend. You don't make deals that compromise yourself or your team, of course, but you help other riders if you can, so they might return the favor.

The politics could be ambiguous and confusing to a young rider, even upsetting, and I got a harsh lesson in them in early 1991. My plan was to race as an amateur through the 1992 Olympics in Barcelona, and to turn pro right afterward. In the meantime, I continued to race in the U.S. for Subaru–Montgomery. Technically, I was a member of two different teams: internationally, I raced for the U.S. national team under Chris Carmichael, but domestically I competed for Subaru–Montgomery.

While I was overseas with the national team in '91, we entered a prestigious race in Italy called the Settimana Bergamasca. It was a pro-am stage race, a ten-day ride through northern Italy, and some of the best cyclists in the world would be there. No American had ever won it—but our U.S. team under Chris had great morale and teamwork, and we felt we might just pull it off.

There was an awkwardness, however. The Subaru–Montgomery team was also entered, and I would be racing against them, riding in my stars and stripes, while they would wear their Subaru–Montgomery jerseys. Nine days out of ten, they were my teammates, but for this race, we would be competitors.

Early in the race, a Subaru–Montgomery rider and friend of mine, Nate Reese, took the overall lead. But I was riding well, too. I moved into second. I was exultant; it seemed like the best of both worlds to have the two of us riding at the front. But the Subaru–Montgomery team director didn't feel the same way. He was not happy to see me in contention, and he let me know it. Between two stages, he called me over. "You work for Nate," he said to me. I stared at him, uncomprehending. Surely he didn't mean I was supposed to hang back and play the role of domestique to Nate? But that's exactly what he did mean. "You're not to attack," he ordered. Then he told me straight out that I was obliged to let Nate win.

I was deeply loyal to the national team. Compared to the rest of the field, we were underdogs, a ragtag crew staying in a tiny hotel, three guys to a room, with no money. We were on such a tight budget that Chris washed our water bottles each night and recycled them, while the pro teams like Subaru–Montgomery would throw theirs away after one use. If I could win the Settimana Bergamasca, it would be a huge victory for the U.S. program, and for American cycling in general. But my trade-team manager was telling me to hold back.

I went to Chris and confessed that I was being told not to ride hard by the Subaru–Montgomery director. "Lance, this is your race to win," Chris said. "You *can't* not attack. It's yours."

The next day, I rode hard. Imagine: you're going up a hill with 100 guys in the peloton. Gradually, 50 guys get dropped, then 20 more get dropped, and then 10 more. You're down to 15 or 20 guys. It's a race of attrition. To make things even harder on your competitors, you attack—raise the tempo even more. Those remaining riders who can't keep up get dropped, too. That's the essence of road racing.

But I was supposed to wait for Nate. The more I thought about it, it was not even an option. I said to myself, *If he's strong enough to stay here, fine. If he gets dropped, I'm not waiting for him.* He got dropped. And I didn't wait for him.

I went with the leaders, and at the end of the day I wore the leader's jersey, while Nate had lost about 20 minutes or so. The Subaru–Montgomery team director was furious, and afterward, he angrily confronted Chris and me. "What are you trying to do?" he asked. Chris jumped to my defense.

"Hey, this is a bike race," Chris said. "He's riding to win."

As we walked away, I was deeply upset. On the one hand I felt betrayed and abandoned by the team director, and on the other, I still struggled with guilt and conflicting loyalty. That night, Chris and I sat down to talk again. "Look, if people are saying you shouldn't attack, they aren't thinking about what's best for you," Chris said. "This is a historic race and an American has never won it, and you're riding it with the best pros in Italy. If you win, it's great for your career. What's more, you're riding for the U.S. national team. If you don't do your best, what message does that send?"

In my opinion, it would have been the worst possible message: "Sorry I'm in the lead—I have to let this other guy win because he's a pro." I couldn't do it. Yet I was worried that the team director could damage my future as a pro by bad-mouthing me.

Chris said, "Don't worry, you just do what you think is right. If you win this race, you're going to be set."

I wanted to talk to my mother. I could barely figure out the phones and how to dial the States, but I finally got through to her.

"Son, what's going on?" she said.

I explained the situation, so upset I was practically stuttering. "Mom, I don't know what to do," I said. "I'm in one of the leading positions, but the Subaru director is telling me Nate Reese is going to win, and I have to help him."

My mother listened, and then she said, "Lance, if you feel like you can win the race, you do it."

"I think I can."

"Then to hell with them," she said. "You're going to win this race. Don't let anybody intimidate you—you put your head down, and you race."

I put my head down, and I raced. I was an unpopular leader, and not just with Subaru–Montgomery; the Italian race fans lining the course were so incensed that an American was in front that they scattered glass and thumbtacks in the road, hoping I would blow a tire. But as the race wore on, the Italians steadily warmed to me, and by the time I crossed the finish line, they cheered.

I was the winner. I had done it, given the U.S. national team a victory in a European race. Our team was ecstatic, and so was Chris. That night, as I came down from the podium, Chris told me something I've never forgotten.

"You're gonna win the Tour de France one day," he said.

CYCLING IS A SPORT THAT EMBARRASSES YOUTH, rather than rewards it. As I had planned, I turned pro immediately after the Olympics—and immediately finished dead last in my very first race.

I'd had a disappointing performance in the Barcelona Games, finishing 14th in the road race, but somehow I managed to impress one of the most influential men in American cycling, a man named Jim Ochowicz, who took a chance and signed me to a pro contract. "Och," as everybody called him, was the director of a team sponsored by Motorola, made up primarily of American riders. Och was a cycling pioneer: in 1985 he had organized the first predominantly American squad to race overseas, and proven that U.S. riders could compete in the traditionally European sport.(One of those early riders for Och's Team 7-Eleven was Chris Carmichael.) A year later, Greg LeMond won the 1986 Tour de France and brought the event into the American consciousness.

Och was always on the lookout for rising young Americans, and Chris steered me toward him. He introduced us one night in the midst of the Tour Du Pont, the biggest stage race held on American soil. I went to Och's hotel for what amounted to a job interview. I didn't realize it then, but I was meeting my surrogate father.

My first impression was of a gangly, soft-spoken man in his 40s with an easy laugh and a broad, toothy smile. We sat around and chatted about where I came from, and he told me what he was looking for in a rider: he wanted to find a young American who might follow in LeMond's footsteps and win the Tour de France. Och's teams had placed riders fourth on a couple of different occasions, but had never won it.

Och asked me what my own ambition was. "I want to be the best rider there is," I said. "I want to go to Europe and be a pro. I don't want to just be good at it, I want to be the best." That was good enough for Och; he handed me a contract and packed me off to Europe.

My first race was the Clásica San Sebastián. They may call it a "classic," but in reality it's a horribly punishing single-day race in which riders cover more than a hundred miles, frequently over bone-rattling terrain, in terrible weather. It is atmospheric and historic, and notoriously brutal. San Sebastián turned out to be a gorgeous seaside town in Basque country, but the day of my debut was gray, pouring rain, and bitingly cold. There is nothing more uncomfortable than riding in the rain, because you can never, ever get warm. Your Lycra jersey is nothing more than a second skin. Cold rain soaks it, plastering it to your body, so the chill mingles with your sweat and seeps down into your bones. Your muscles seize up and grow heavy with frigid, sodden exhaustion.

The day of my debut, it rained so hard it hurt. As we started off into the stinging, icy downpour, I quickly faded to the back, and as the day wore on, I slipped farther and farther behind, shivering and struggling to pedal. Soon, I was in last place. Ahead of me, the field was growing thinner as riders began to give up. Every so often one would pull over to the side of the road and abandon the race. I was tempted to do the same, to squeeze the brakes, rise up from the bars, and coast to the side of the road. It would be so easy. But I couldn't, not in my first pro start. It would be too humiliating. What would my teammates think? I wasn't a quitter.

Why don't you just quit?

Son, you never quit.

Fifty riders dropped out, but I kept pedaling. I came in dead last in the field of 111 riders. I crossed the finish line almost half an hour behind the winner, and as I churned up the last hill, the Spanish crowd began to laugh and hiss at me. "Look at the sorry one in last place," one jeered.

A few hours later, I sat in the Madrid airport, slumped in a chair. I wanted to quit the entire sport. It was the most sobering race of my life; on my way to San Sebastián, I had actually thought I had a chance of winning, and now I wondered if I could compete at all. They had laughed at me.

Professional cycling was going to be a lot harder than I'd thought; the pace was faster, the terrain tougher, the competition more fit than I ever imagined. I pulled a sheaf of unused plane tickets out of my pocket. Among them, I had a return portion to the States. I considered using it. *Maybe I should just go home,* I thought, and find something else to do, something I was good at.

I went to a pay phone and called Chris Carmichael. I told him how depressed I was, and that I was considering quitting. Chris just listened, and then he said, "Lance, you are going to learn more from that experience than any other race in your whole life." I was right to have stayed in and finished, to prove to my new teammates that I was a tough rider. If they were going to rely on me, they needed to know I wasn't a quitter. Now they did.

"Okay," I said. "Okay. I'll keep going."

I hung up, and boarded the plane for the next race. I had just two days off, and then I was scheduled to compete in the Championship of Zurich. I had a lot to prove, to myself and everyone else—and unless my heart exploded in my chest, I was not going to be last again.

I finished second in Zurich. I attacked from the start and stayed on the attack for practically the entire race. I had little or no idea tactically how to ride in the race—I just put my head down and bulled through it, and when I stepped onto the medal podium it was more with relief than elation. *Okay,* I thought to myself, *I think I can do this after all.*

I called Chris Carmichael. "See?" Chris said. In the space of just a few days I had gone from depressed rookie to legitimate competitor. The turnaround provoked murmurs around the sport: *Who's this guy and what's he all about?* people wanted to know.

It was a question I still needed to answer for myself.

AN AMERICAN IN CYCLING WAS COMPARABLE TO A French baseball team in the World Series. I was a gate-crasher in a revered and time-honored sport, and I had little or no concept of its rules, written and unwritten, or its etiquette. Let's just say that my Texas manners didn't exactly play well on the continent.

There was a big difference between the discreet jockeying of European cycling, and the swaggering, trash-talking American idea of competition I was reared with. Like most Americans, I grew up oblivious to cycling; it wasn't until LeMond's victory in the '86 Tour that I really noticed the sport. There was a way things were done, and attitudes that I didn't understand, and even when I did understand them I didn't feel I had to be a part of them. In fact, I ignored them.

I raced with no respect. Absolutely none. I paraded, mouthed off, shoved my fists in the air. I never backed down. The journalists loved me; I was different, I made good copy, I was colorful. But I was making enemies.

A road is only so wide. Riders are constantly moving around, fighting for position, and often the smart and diplomatic thing to do is to let a fellow rider in. In a long stage race, you give a little to make a friend, because you might need one later. Give an inch, make a friend. But I wouldn't do it. Partly it was my character at the time: I was insecure and defensive, not totally confident of how strong I was. I was still the kid from Plano with the chip on my shoulder, riding headlong, pedaling out of anger. I didn't think I could afford to give up inches.

Sometimes I would yell at other riders in the peloton, in frustration: "Pull or get out of the way!" I didn't understand yet that for various reasons a guy might sit on the back, maybe because his team leader told him to, or because he was tired and hurting. It wasn't his job to move out of my way, or to work harder so I could ride at a faster pace. (I don't get so riled up about those things anymore, and often I'm the one who sits on the back, hurting.)

I would learn that in the peloton, other riders can totally mess you up, just to keep you from winning. There is a term in cycling, "flicking." It's a derivative of the German word *ficken,* which means "to fuck." If you flick somebody in the peloton, it means to screw him, just to get him. There's a lot of flicking in the peloton.

Guys would flick me just to flick me. They would race to see that I didn't win, simply because they didn't like me. They could cut me off. They could isolate me, and make me ride slower, or they could surge and push the pace, making me work harder than I wanted to, weakening me. Fortunately I was surrounded by some protective teammates, guys like Sean Yates, Steve Bauer, and Frankie Andreu, who tried to gently explain that I wasn't doing myself any good, or them either. "Lance, you've got to try to control yourself, you're making enemies," Frankie would say. They seemed to understand that I had some maturing to do, and if they were exasperated with me, they kept it to themselves, and patiently steered me in the right direction.

Teammates are critical in cycling—I had eight of them on the Motorola squad, and I needed each and every one. On a severe climb it could save me thirty percent of my energy to ride behind a colleague, drafting, "sitting on his wheel." Or, on a windy day, my eight teammates would stay out in front of me, shielding me and saving me up to 50 percent of the work I'd have to do otherwise. Every team needs guys who are sprinters, guys who are climbers, guys willing to do the dirty work. It was very important to recognize the effort of each person involved—and not to waste it. "Who's going to work hard for someone who doesn't win?" Och asked me, and it was a good question.

You don't win a road race all on your own. You need your teammates—and you need the goodwill and cooperation of your competitors, too. People had to *want* to ride for you, and with you. But in those first months, a couple of my competitors literally wanted to punch me out.

I would insult great European champions. In one of my first races as a pro, the Tour of the Mediterranean, I encountered Moreno Argentin, a very serious, very respected Italian cyclist. He was one of the dons of the sport, a former World Champion who had won races all over the continent. But I surged right up to the front and challenged him. There were 150 guys bunched all together, jockeying for position, flicking, coming over on each other, and pushing each other out of the way.

As I drew even with Argentin, he glanced at me, vaguely surprised, and said, "What are you doing here, Bishop?"

For some reason it infuriated me. He didn't know my name. He thought I was Andy Bishop, another member of the American team. I thought, *This guy doesn't know my name?*

"Fuck you, Chiapucci!" I said, calling him by the name of one of his teammates.

Argentin did a double take, incredulous. He was the *capo,* the boss, and to him I was a faceless young American who had yet to win anything, yet here I was cussing him out. But I'd had a number of promising results, and in my own mind, he should have known who I was.

"Hey, Chiapucci," I said. "My name's Lance Armstrong, and by the end of this race you'll know it."

For the rest of the race, my sole aim was to throw Argentin off his pedestal headfirst. But in the end, I faded. It was a five-day stage race, and I couldn't keep up—I was too inexperienced. Afterward, Argentin came to our team compound, screaming. He ranted at my teammates about my behavior. That was part of the etiquette too; if a young rider was becoming a problem, it was up to the older riders to get him in line. Roughly translated, what Argentin was saying was, "You need to teach him some manners."

A few days later, I entered a race in Italy, this one the Trophée Laigueglia, a one-day classic. The Trophée was considered an automatic win for Argentin, and I knew it. The favorites in any race in Italy were, of course, the Italians, and especially their leader Argentin. One thing you didn't do to a veteran cyclist was disrespect him in his home country, in front of his fans and sponsors. But I went after him again. I challenged him when nobody else would, and this time the result was different. In the Trophée Laigueglia, I won the duel.

At the end of the race, it was a breakaway of four riders, and at the front were Argentin, Chiapucci, a Venezuelan named Sierra—and me. I hurled myself through the final sprint, and took the lead. Argentin couldn't believe he was going to lose to me, the loudmouth American.

He then did something that has always stayed with me. Five yards from the finish line, he braked. He locked up his wheels—intentionally. He took fourth, out of the medals. I won the race.

There are three places on a podium, and Argentin didn't want to stand beside me. In an odd way, it made more of an impression on me than any lecture or fistfight could have. What he was saying was that he didn't respect me. It was a curiously elegant form of insult, and an effective one.

In the years since then, I've grown up and learned to admire things Italian: their exquisite manners, art, food, and articulacy, not to mention their great rider, Moreno Argentin. In fact, Argentin and I have become good friends. I have a great deal of affection for him, and when we see each other these days, we embrace, Italian style, and laugh.

MY RESULTS CONTINUED TO VEER UP AND DOWN, AS crazily as I wove through a peloton. I'd attack anytime. I'd just go. Someone would surge, and I'd counter, not out of any sense of real strategy, but as if to say, "Is that all you got?"

I had my share of results because I was a strong kid, and I rode on the tactics and coattails of others, but much of the time I was too aggressive, repeating the same critical mistake I'd made riding for Chris Carmichael back in Japan: I'd charge to the front and ride all by myself, and then falter. Sometimes I didn't even finish in the top 20. Afterward one of my teammates would ask, "What the hell were you doing?"

"I felt good," I'd say, lamely.

But I was fortunate to ride for two very smart, sensitive coaches: I continued to train with Chris as part of the national team, while Och and his team director, Henny Kuiper, managed my daily racing for

Motorola. They spent a lot of time on the phone comparing notes, and they recognized and agreed on something important: my strength was the sort you couldn't teach or train. You can teach someone how to control their strength, but you can't teach them to be strong.

While my aggression wasn't winning me friends in the peloton, it might become a valuable asset one day, they suspected. Och and Chris felt that endurance events were not only about suffering pain, but about inflicting it, too, and in my attacking nature they saw the beginnings of something predatory. "You ever hear about how when you stab somebody, it's really personal?" Chris said once. "Well, a bike race is that kind of personal. Don't kid yourself. It's a knife fight."

Och and Chris felt that if I ever gained control of my temperament, I'd be a rider to reckon with. In the meantime they handled me very carefully, intuiting that if they started yelling at me, I would most likely turn off, or rebel. They decided the lessons should sink in slowly.

There are some things you learn better through experience, and Och and Chris let me figure it out on my own. At first, I never evaluated my races. I'd think, "I was the strongest rider out there; those guys couldn't keep up with me." But when I lost several races, I was forced to think again, and one day it finally occurred to me: "Wait a minute. If I'm the strongest guy, why didn't I win?"

Slowly, steadily, Och and Chris passed along their knowledge of the character of various courses, and the way a race evolves tactically. "There are moments when you can use your energy to your benefit, and there are moments when you use it to no avail. That's a waste," Och said.

I began to listen to the other riders, and let them rein me in. I roomed with two veterans, Sean Yates and Steve Bauer, who had a lot of influence over me. I fed off them, picked up a lot of knowledge just sitting around the dinner table. They helped to keep my feet on the ground. I was Mr. Energy, bouncing off the walls, saying things like, "Let's go out there and kick butt!" They would roll their eyes.

Och not only tamed me; more important, he educated me. I was uncomfortable living in Europe seven months out the year; I missed my Shiner Bock beer and Mexican food, I missed the hot, dry Texas fields, and I missed my apartment in Austin, where I had a longhorn skull over the fireplace mantel covered in red, white, and blue leather, with a Lone Star on his forehead. I whined about the cars, the hotels, the food. "Why are we staying at this dump?" I'd say. I was learning a cycling tradition: the discomfort of the sport extends to the accommodations. Some of the hotels we stayed in made Motel 6 look pretty nice—there were crumbs on the bare floors and hairs in the bedsheets. To me, the meat was mysterious, the pasta was soggy, and the coffee tasted like brown water. But eventually I became acclimated, and thanks to my teammates, my discomfort got to be funny. We'd pull up in front of our next hotel, and they'd just wait for me to start complaining.

When I look back at the raw young rider and person I was, I feel impatience with him, but I also feel some sympathy. Underneath the tough talk and the combativeness and the bitching, I was afraid. I was afraid of everything. I was afraid of the train schedules and the airports and the roads. I was afraid of the phones, because I didn't know how to dial them. I was afraid of the menus, because I couldn't read them.

Once, at a dinner for some Japanese business executives hosted by Och, I particularly distinguished myself. Och asked that each of the riders introduce himself, stating his name and country. I stood up. "Hello, I'm Lance from Texas," I boomed. The whole party broke up. They were laughing at me again.

But inevitably, living in Europe began to polish me. I rented an apartment in Lake Como, Italy, and was charmed by that misty, dusty town tucked in the Italian Alps. Och was a wine lover, and I benefited from his taste, learning to recognize fine food and fine wine. I discovered I had a knack for languages. I was beginning to speak bits of Spanish, Italian, and French, and I could even limp around in Dutch if I had to. I window-shopped through Milan, where I learned what a really handsome suit looked like. One afternoon I walked into the Duomo, and in that instant all of my ideas about art changed forever. I was overwhelmed by the color and proportion of it, by the gray stillness in the archways, the warm parchment glow of the candles and the soaring stained glass, the eloquence of the sculptures.

As the summer approached, I was growing up. On the bike, things began to come together and my riding steadied. "It's all happening," Och said. And it was. An American race sponsor, Thrift Drugs, put up a $1 million bonus for anyone who could win the Triple Crown of Cycling, a sweep of three prestigious races in the U.S. I fixated on it. Each race was different: to get the bonus you'd have to win a tough one-day race in Pittsburgh, then a six-day stage race in West Virginia, and finally the U.S. Pro Championships, which was a one-day road race covering 156 miles through Philadelphia. It was a long shot, the promoters knew. Only a complete rider could win it: you'd have to be a sprinter, a climber, and a stage racer rolled into one, and most important, you'd have to be thoroughly consistent—something I hadn't yet been.

All the riders talked about winning the bonus, and in the next breath we'd talk about how impossible it was. But one night when I was on the phone with my mother she asked me, "What are the odds of winning that thing?"

I said, "Good."

By June I had won the first two legs, and the press was going crazy and the promoters were reeling. All that remained was the U.S. Pro Championships in Philly—but I would have 119 other cyclists trying to stop me. The anticipation was huge; an estimated half a million people would line the route.

The day before the race I called my mother and asked her to fly up to Philadelphia. On such short notice, she'd have to pay almost $1,000 round-trip, but she decided it was like buying a lottery ticket—if she didn't come, and I won, she'd always regret not being there.

I was resolved to ride a smart race, no irrational headfirst charges. *Think the race through,* I told myself.

For most of the day, that's what I did. Then, with about 20 miles left, I went. I attacked on the most notoriously steep part of the course—Manayunk—and as I did, I was almost in a rage. I don't know what happened—all I know is that I leaped out of the seat and hammered down on the pedals, and as I did so I screamed for five full seconds. I opened up a huge gap on the field.

By the second-to-last lap, I had enough of a lead to blow my mother a kiss. I crossed the finish line with the biggest winning margin in race history. I dismounted in a swarm of reporters, but I broke away from them and went straight to my mom, and we put our faces in each other's shoulder and cried.

That was the start of a dreamlike summer season. Next, I won a surprise victory in a stage of the Tour de France with another late charge: at the end of a 114-mile ride from Châlons-sur-Marne to Verdun, I nearly crashed into the race barriers as I sprinted away from the pack over the last 50 yards to the finish. A Tour stage was considered an extremely valuable victory in its own right, and at 21, I was the youngest man ever to win one.

But to show you just how experienced you have to be to compete in the Tour, I had to pull out of the race a couple of days later, incapable of continuing. I abandoned after the 12th stage, in 97th place and shivering. The Alps got me; they were "too long and too cold," I told reporters afterward. I fell so far behind that when I got to the finish line, the team car had already left for the hotel. I had to walk back to our rooms, pushing my bike up a gravel trail. "As if the stage wasn't enough, we have to climb this thing," I told the press. I wasn't physically mature enough yet to ride the arduous mountain stages.

I still struggled with impatience at times. I would ride smart for a while, and then backslide. I just couldn't seem to get it through my head that in order to win I had to ride more slowly at first. It took some time to reconcile myself to the notion that being patient was different from being weak, and that racing strategically didn't mean giving less than all I had.

With only a week to go before the World Championships, I made a typical blunder in the championship of Zurich and used myself up before the critical part of the race. Again, I didn't even finish in the Top 20. Och could have lost his temper with me; instead he stayed over in Zurich for the next two days and went riding with me. He was certain I could win at the Worlds in Oslo—but only if I rode intelligently. As we trained together he chatted to me about self-control.

"The only thing you have to do is wait," he said. "Just *wait*. Two or three laps is soon enough. Anything earlier and you'll waste your chance to win. But after that, you can attack as many times as you want."

There were no ordinary cyclists in the World Championships. I would be facing big riders, at their peak, and the favorite was Miguel Indurain, who had just come off of his third victory in the Tour de France. If I wanted to win I'd have to overcome some long historical odds; no 21-year-old had ever won a world title in cycling.

In the last few days leading up to the race, I called my mother again, and asked her to come over and stay with me. I didn't want to go through it alone, and she had always been a source of confidence for me. Also, I wanted her to see me race in that company. She took some vacation time from Ericsson and flew over to join me, and stayed with me in my hotel room.

She took care of me, the way she used to. She did my laundry in the sink, saw that I had what I wanted to eat, answered the phone, and made sure I got my rest. I didn't have to talk cycling with her, or explain how I felt—she just understood. The closer we got to that day, the quieter I grew. I shut down, planning the race in my mind. She just read by a small lamp while I stared at the ceiling or napped.

Finally race day arrived—but when I awoke, it was raining. I opened my eyes and saw drops on the windowpanes. The hated, dreaded rain, the source of so much anguish and embarrassment in San Sebastián.

It rained torrentially, all day long. But there was one person who suffered in the rain more than I did that day: my mother. She sat in a grandstand in the rain for seven hours, and never once got up. There was a big screen mounted in front of the grandstand so the crowd could watch us out on the 18.4-kilometer course, and she sat there, drenched, watching riders crash all over the course.

When it rains in Europe the roads become covered with a slick sort of residue, made of dust and petrol. Guys were thrown off their bikes right and left, their wheels sliding out from under them. I crashed, too, twice. But each time I recovered quickly, got back on the bike, and rejoined the race, still in contention.

Through it all, I waited, and waited. I held back, just as Och had told me to. With 14 laps to go, I was in the lead group—and right there was Indurain, the bravura rider from Spain. Finally, on the second-to-last climb, I attacked. I charged up the hill and reached the peak with my wheel in front of the pack. I hurtled down the descent, and then soared right into another climb, a steep ascent called the Ekeberg, with the other riders right on my back. I said to myself, "I've got to go right now, with everything I've ever gone with," and I rose from the seat and attacked again, and this time I opened up a gap.

On the other side of the Ekeberg was another long, dangerous descent, this one of four kilometers, and in the rain anything could happen; the wheels could disappear out from under you as the entire road became a slick. But I took the turns hard and tight, and at the bottom, I glanced over my shoulder to see who was still with me.

No one.

I panicked. *You made the same old mistake,* I thought, desperately, *you went too early.* I must have forgotten what lap it was. Surely there was still a lap to go, because a lead like this was too good to be true.

I glanced down and checked my computer. It was the last lap.

I was going to win.

Over the last 700 meters, I started celebrating. I pumped my fists and my arms in the air, I blew kisses, and I bowed to the crowd. As I crossed the finish line, I practically high-kicked like a Rockette. Finally, I braked and dismounted, and in the crowds of people, the first thing I did was look for my mother. I found her, and we stood there in the rain, hugging. I said, "We did it! We did it." We both began to cry.

At some point in all of the post-race confusion and celebration and ceremony, a royal escort arrived to inform me that King Harald of Norway wanted to greet me. I nodded and said, "Come on, Mom. Let's go meet the king."

She said, "Well, okay."

We began to move through the security checkpoints. Finally, we approached a door, behind which the king was waiting to give me a private audience. A security guard stopped us. "She'll have to stop here," the royal escort told us. "The king will greet you alone."

"I don't check my mother at the door," I said.

I grabbed her arm and turned around to leave. "Come on, let's go," I said. I had no intention of going anywhere without her.

The escort relented. "All right. Please, come with me." And we met the king, who was a very nice man. Our audience was very short, and polite, and then we went back to celebrating.

It seemed like the end of something for my mother and me, a finish line. The tough part of the fight was over; there would be no more naysayers telling us we wouldn't amount to anything, no more concerns about bills or scrabbling for equipment and plane tickets. Maybe it was the end of the long, hard climb of childhood.

Although I was a world champion, I still had plenty of learning to do, and the next three years were a process of testing and refinement. I had other successes, but life from now on would be a matter of incremental improvements, of seeking the tiniest margin that might separate me from the other elite riders.

There was a science to winning. The spectator rarely sees the technical side of cycling, but behind the gorgeous rainbow blur of the peloton is the more boring reality that road racing is a carefully calibrated thing, and often a race is won by a mere fraction of acceleration that was generated in a performance lab or a wind tunnel or a velodrome long before the race ever started. Cyclists are computer slaves; we hover over precise calculations of cadence, efficiency, force, and wattage. I was constantly sitting on a stationary bike with electrodes all over my body, looking for different positions on the bike that might gain mere seconds, or a piece of equipment that might be a little bit more aerodynamic.

Just a few weeks after winning the Worlds, I went into a performance lab at the Olympic Training Center in Colorado Springs with Chris Carmichael. Despite my big year I still had some critical weaknesses, and I spent several days in the lab, plastered with electrodes while doctors jabbed me with pins for blood tests. The idea was to de-

termine my various thresholds and breaking points, and thus to figure
out how I could increase my efficiency on the bike. They looked at my
heart rate, my VO_2 max, and in one day alone, they pricked my thumb
15 times to check my blood.

We wanted to determine what my maximum effort was, and how
long I could sustain it. We set out to learn my optimum cadence: what
was my most efficient pedal speed, and where were the weaknesses in
my pedaling technique, the dead spots where I was wasting energy?
My stroke was a symmetrical sledgehammer, straight up and down, and
I was expending too much work without getting enough speed from
it. We went into a velodrome to look at my position on the bike and
determine where I was losing power. The idea in cycling is to gener-
ate the most speed with the least amount of work; watts indicate the
amount of work you are doing as you pedal. We shifted me lower on
the bike, and there was an immediate improvement.

At about the same time, I met the legendary Belgian rider Eddy
Merckx, five-time winner of the Tour de France, and one of the most
ferociously attacking riders who's ever lived. I had heard all the stories
about Merckx, what a brave, hard-charging rider he was, and I thought
that was the kind of rider I wanted to be. I didn't just want to win, I
wanted to win a certain way. We became friends. Eddy told me that I
could win a Tour de France someday—but that I needed to lose
weight. I was built like a linebacker, with a thick neck and slabs of
muscle in my chest, remnants of my career as a swimmer and triathlete. Eddy explained that it was hard to haul all of that weight up and
down mountains over three weeks. I was still racing partly on raw
power; to win a Tour de France, I would have to find a way to lose
weight without losing strength. So I quit eating pastry, and laid off Tex-
Mex, and understood that I would have to find a new kind of strength,
that inner strength called self-discipline.

By 1995, I still had not completed an entire Tour de France, only portions. My coaches didn't think I was ready, and they were right; I had neither the body nor the mental toughness yet to endure the hardship. A young rider has to be carefully walked through the process and developed over years until he is ready to finish the race, and finish it healthy. I was steadily improving: in '94 I was second in Liège-Bastogne-Liège, second in San Sebastián, and second in the Tour Du Pont, and in the first part of '95 I won San Sebastián and won the Tour Du Pont. But now Och felt I needed to move to another level, I needed to *finish* the Tour de France, not just start it. It was time for me to learn exactly what it took to win the biggest stage race in the world.

My reputation was as a single-day racer: show me the start line and I would win on adrenaline and anger, chopping off my competitors one by one. I could push myself to a threshold of pain no one else was willing to match, and I would bite somebody's head off to win a race.

But the Tour was another thing entirely. If you raced that way in the Tour, you would have to drop out after two days. It required a longer view. The Tour was a matter of mustering the right resources at the right times, of patiently feeding out your strength at the necessary level, with no wasted motion or energy. It was a matter of continuing to ride and ride, no matter how uninspired you felt, when there was no rush of adrenaline left to push you.

If there is a defining characteristic of a man as opposed to a boy, maybe it's patience. In 1995, I finally gained an understanding of the demanding nature of the Tour and all of its extraordinary tests and dangers. I finished it, and I finished strong, winning a stage in the closing days. But the knowledge came at too high a price, and I would just as soon not have learned it the way I did.

Late in the race, our Motorola teammate, Fabio Casartelli, the 1992 Olympic champion, was killed on a high-speed descent. On a descent, you ride single file, and if one rider goes down, it can cause a terrible chain reaction. Fabio didn't crash alone; 20 riders went down with him. But he hit a curb with the back of his head and fractured his neck and skull.

I went by too fast to see much. A lot of riders were down, and everybody was crouched around someone lying on the ground, but you see that sort of thing a lot in the Tour. It was only a while later that I learned via the team radio what had happened: Fabio was dead. When they tell you something like that, you almost don't believe it.

It was one of the longest days of my life. Fabio was not only the young hope of Italian cycling, he was a new husband and a new father. His baby was just a month old.

We had to keep riding, to finish the stage even though we were distraught and sick with shock. I had known Fabio since I first started racing internationally in '91. He lived right outside of Como where I kept my apartment, and we had competed against each other at the Barcelona Olympics in '92, when he won the gold medal. He was a very relaxed, fun-loving man, a little goofy, a joker. Some of the top Italians were more serious, or macho, but Fabio wasn't like that. He was all sweetness.

That night we had a Motorola team meeting to discuss whether we should keep riding or not. We were split. Half of us wanted to quit and go home and cry with our families and friends, and half of us wanted to keep riding in honor of Fabio. Personally, I wanted to stop; I simply didn't think I had the heart to ride a bike. It was the first time I had encountered death, and genuine grief, and I didn't know how to handle it. But then Fabio's wife came to see us, and she said she wanted us to keep riding, because she felt that was what Fabio would have wanted. So we sat in the grass behind the hotel, said a few prayers, and decided to stay in.

The next day the peloton rode in honor of Fabio, and gave our team a ceremonial stage victory. It was another long, terrible day—eight hours on the bike, with everybody grieving. The peloton did not race. Instead we rode in quiet formation. It was virtually a funeral procession, and at last our team rode across the finish line, while, behind us, Fabio's bike was mounted atop the support car with a black ribbon.

The following morning we began the race again in earnest, and rode into Bordeaux. Next was a stage into Limoges, and that night, Och came around to our rooms and told the team that Fabio had had two goals in the Tour: he wanted to finish the race, and he especially wanted to try to win the stage into Limoges. As soon as Och stopped speaking I knew that if Limoges was the stage Fabio had wanted to win for himself, now I wanted to win it for him, and that I was going to finish the race.

About halfway through the next day's stage, I found myself grouped with 25 guys at the front. Indurain was in the yellow leader's jersey, riding at the back. I did what came most naturally to me: I attacked.

The problem was, I attacked too early, as usual. I went with 25 miles still to go, and on a downhill portion. Two things you never do: attack early, and on a downhill. But I went so fast on that downhill that I had a 30-second lead in a finger-snap. The other riders were completely taken aback. I could feel them wondering, *What's he thinking?*

What was I thinking? I had looked back, and saw guys were riding along, with no particular ambition. It was a hot day, and there was no incentive to pull hard, everyone was just trying to get closer to the finish line where the tactics would play out. I glanced back, and one guy was taking a sip of water. I glanced back again. Another guy was fixing his hat. So I took off. *Peoooo.* I was gone.

When you have 15 other guys back there from 15 different teams, they'll never get organized. They'll look at each other and say: *You pull. No, you pull!* So I went, and I went faster than I'd ever ridden. It was a tactical punch in the face, and it had nothing to do with strength or ability; everything depended on the initial shock and separation. It was insane, but it worked.

Nobody got within 55 seconds of me again. The team support car kept coming up and giving me reports. Henny Kuiper, our team director, would say, "You're thirty seconds up." Then a few minutes later he'd come alongside again and say, "You're forty-five seconds up."

When he came up the third or fourth time, I said, "Henny, don't come up here anymore. I'm not getting caught."

"Okay, okay, okay," he said, and faded behind my wheel.

I didn't get caught.

I won by a minute, and I didn't feel a moment's pain. Instead I felt something spiritual; I know that I rode with a higher purpose that day. Even though I had charged too early, I never suffered after I broke away. I would like to think that was Fabio's experience too; he simply broke away and separated from the world. There is no doubt in my mind that there were two riders on that bike. Fabio was with me.

I felt an emotion at the finish line that I've never experienced again. I felt I was winning for Fabio and his family and his baby, and for the mourning country of Italy. As I came across the line I glanced upward and I pointed to the heavens, to Fabio.

After the Tour, Och had a memorial built for Fabio. He commissioned a sculptor from Como to execute a work in white Carrara marble. The team flew in from all over the world, and we gathered at the top of the mountain for the placement of the memorial and the dedication ceremony. The memorial had a sundial on it that shone on three dates and times: his birthday, the day he won the Olympic Games, and the day he died.

I had learned what it means to ride the Tour de France. It's not about the bike. It's a metaphor for life, not only the longest race in the world but also the most exalting and heartbreaking and potentially tragic. It poses every conceivable element to the rider, and more: cold, heat, mountains, plains, ruts, flat tires, high winds, unspeakably bad luck, unthinkable beauty, yawning senselessness, and above all a great, deep self-questioning. During our lives we're faced with so many different elements as well, we experience so many setbacks, and fight such a hand-to-hand battle with failure, head down in the rain, just trying to stay upright and to have a little hope. The Tour is not just a bike race, not at all. It is a test. It tests you physically, it tests you mentally, and it even tests you morally.

I understood that now. There were no shortcuts, I realized. It took years of racing to build up the mind and body and character, until a rider had logged hundreds of races and thousands of miles of road. I wouldn't be able to win a Tour de France until I had enough iron in my legs, and lungs, and brain, and heart. Until I was a man. Fabio had been a man. I was still trying to get there.

four

BAD TO WORSE

I THOUGHT I KNEW WHAT FEAR WAS, UNTIL I heard the words *You have cancer.* Real fear came with an unmistakable sensation: it was as though all my blood started flowing in the wrong direction. My previous fears, fear of not being liked, fear of being laughed at, fear of losing my money, suddenly seemed like small cowardices. Everything now stacked up differently: the anxieties of life— a flat tire, losing my career, a traffic jam—were reprioritized into need versus want, real problem as opposed to minor scare. A bumpy plane ride was just a bumpy plane ride, it wasn't cancer.

One definition of "human" is as follows: *characteristic of people as opposed to God or animals or machines, especially susceptible to weakness, and therefore showing the qualities of man.* Athletes don't tend to think of themselves in these terms; they're too busy cultivating the aura of invincibility to admit to being fearful, weak, defenseless, vulnerable, or fallible, and for that reason neither are they especially kind, considerate, merciful, benign, lenient, or forgiving, to themselves or anyone around them. But as I sat in my house alone that first night, it was humbling to be so scared. More than that, it was humanizing.

I wasn't strong enough to break it to my mother that I was sick. Not long after I arrived home from Dr. Reeves' office, Rick Parker came over because he didn't think I should be alone. I told Rick that I simply couldn't bear to call my mother with the news. "I don't want to tell her," I said. Rick offered to do it for me, and I accepted.

There was no gentle way to say it. She had just gotten home from work and was sitting outside in her garden, reading the paper, when the call came. Rick said, "Linda, Lance is going to need to talk to you about this himself, but I just want to let you know what's going on. He's been diagnosed with testicular cancer, and he's having surgery tomorrow at 7 A.M."

My mother said, "No. How can this be?"

Rick said, "I'm sorry, but I think you need to come down here tonight."

My mother began to cry, and Rick tried to comfort her, but he also wanted her to get on a shuttle to Austin as quickly as possible. My mother changed gears. "Okay," she said. "Okay, I'll be right there." She hung up without even speaking with me, and immediately threw whatever she could think of into a small bag and raced to the airport.

After Rick hung up from talking with my mother, I broke down again. Rick calmly talked me through it. "It's natural for you to cry," he said. "It's even good for you. Lance, this is curable. It's a speed bump. We need to get on with whipping this thing."

Shored up, I went into my study and I began to make calls to the other people I felt I needed to tell immediately. I called my friend and

Motorola teammate Kevin Livingston, who was in Europe racing. Kevin was like a younger brother to me; we were so close that we had plans to get an apartment together in Europe the following season, and I had persuaded him to move to Austin to train with me. When I reached him in Italy, I still felt spaced out. "I have something to tell you—something bad has happened."

"What? Did something go wrong with a race?"

"I have cancer."

I wanted to tell Kevin how I felt and how urgently I wanted to see him, but he was in an apartment with three other members of the U.S. national team, and I didn't want them to know. So we had to talk in code.

"You know," I said.

He replied, "Yeah. I know."

And that was it, we got off the phone. The very next day, he was on a plane for home.

Next, I reached Bart Knaggs, perhaps my oldest and best friend in Austin, a former cyclist who was working for a start-up computer-technology company. I found him at his office, where he was working late, like always. "Bart, I have testicular cancer," I said. Bart stammered, not sure what to say, and then he said, "Lance, they do wonders with cancer now, and I think if you have to get it, that's a good one to have."

I said, "I don't know. I'm sitting here alone in my house, man, and I'm really scared."

Bart, typically, entered a search command into his computer, and called up everything there was to know about the disease. He sat there until late, researching testicular cancer, and printed out what he found until he had a pile a foot high. He called up clinical trials, studies, and treatment options, and downloaded it all. Then he gathered it up and drove over to my house. He had to go to Orlando early the following morning with his fiancée, Barbara, but he came by to tell me he loved me, and gave me all of the cancer material.

One by one, my friends and family began to arrive. Lisa came, after I paged her; she had been studying in the library and she was glassy-eyed with shock at the news. Next, Bill Stapleton arrived with his wife, Laura. Bill was a young attorney for a firm in Austin, and I had chosen him to represent me because he exuded loyalty. He was an ambling sort outwardly, but he was a competitor, too, a former Olympic swimmer from the University of Texas who still had the look of an athlete. When he came in, I fixated on what I was sure was the loss of my career.

"I'm done racing," I said. "I won't need an agent anymore."

"Lance, we just need to deal with this one step at a time," Bill said. "You have no idea what this means, or what's going to happen."

"You don't understand, Bill. I'm not going to have an agent anymore. I'm not going to have any contracts."

"Well, I'm not here as an agent, I'm here as your friend. How can I help?"

It was one of those moments when everything shifted. I was obsessing over the fact that I was going to lose my career, when there were more important things to attend to.

"You can pick up my mother at the airport," I said.

Bill and Laura immediately got up from the sofa and drove to the airport to get my mother. I was just as glad not to meet her flight, because as soon as she saw Bill, she broke down in tears again. "This is my baby," she told Bill and Laura. "How could this happen? What are we going to do?" But during the drive to my house, my mother collected herself. She was born without an ounce of self-pity, and by the time she reached my driveway she was strong again. As soon as she walked in the house, I met her in the center of the living room and gave her a bear hug.

"We're going to be okay," my mother said into my ear. "This isn't going to get us. We've had too many things to deal with. This is one thing that won't happen. Don't even try this with me."

We both cried a little then, but not for very long, because there was too much to discuss. I sat down with my friends and my mother, and explained to them what the diagnosis from Dr. Reeves was. There were some issues to go over and some decisions to be made, and we didn't have much time, because I was scheduled for surgery at 7 A.M. I pulled out the X ray that I'd brought home from Dr. Reeves, and showed it to everybody. You could see the tumors, like white golf balls, floating in my lungs.

I was concerned about keeping the illness quiet until I'd had time to tell my sponsors and teammates. While I continued to talk to my mother, Bill called the hospital and asked that my diagnosis be kept confidential and that I be checked in under an assumed name. Also, we had to tell my sponsors, Nike, Giro, Oakley, and Milton-Bradley, as well as the Cofidis organization, and it would be necessary to hold a press conference. But first and foremost I had to tell the people who were closest to me, friends like Och, and Chris, and my teammates, and most of them were scattered overseas and difficult to reach.

Everyone reacted differently to the news; some people stuttered, and some tried to reassure me, but what all of my friends had in common was their urge to come to Austin as quickly as possible. Och was at home in Wisconsin having dinner when I reached him, and his reaction was, in retrospect, pure him.

"Are you sitting down?" I asked.

"What's going on?"

"I've got cancer."

"Okay. What does that mean?"

"It means I've got testicular cancer and I'm having surgery tomorrow."

"All right, let me think about this," Och said, calmly. "I'll see you tomorrow."

Finally, it was time to go to bed. The funny thing was, I slept deeply that night. I went into a state of absolutely perfect rest, as if I was getting ready for a big competition. If I had a tough race in front of me I always made sure to get the optimum amount of sleep, and this was no different, I suppose. On some unconscious level, I wanted to be in absolutely peak form for what I would be faced with in the coming days.

The next morning, I reported to the hospital at 5. I drove myself there, with my mother in the passenger seat, and I walked through the entrance in a baggy sweatsuit to begin life as a cancer patient. First came a series of basic tests, things like MRIs and blood work. I had a faint hope that the doctors would do all their tests and tell me they had been wrong, that my illness wasn't that serious. But those words didn't come.

I had never stayed overnight in a hospital, and I didn't know about things like registration, so I hadn't even brought my wallet. I guess I was always too busy throwing away my crutches and taking out my own stitches. I looked at my mother—and she immediately volunteered to take care of the paperwork. While I was having blood tests done, she filled out the stack of forms the hospital required.

I was in surgery and recovery for about three hours. It seemed like an eternity to my mother, who sat in my hospital room with Bill Stapleton and waited for me to come back. Dr. Reeves came by and told her that it had gone well, they had removed the tumor with no problem. Then Och arrived. True to his word, he had gotten on an early-morning plane for Austin. While I was still in surgery, my mom filled Och in on what was happening. She said she was determined that I was going to be okay, as if the sheer force of her will could make things all right.

Finally, they wheeled me back to my room. I was still foggy from the anesthesia, but I was alert enough to talk to Och as he leaned over my bed. "I'm going to beat this thing, whatever it is," I said.

The hospital kept me overnight, and my mother stayed with me, sleeping on a small sofa. Neither of us rested well. The aftermath of the surgery was very painful—the incision was long and deep and in a tender place, and every time my mother heard my sheets rustle, she would jump up and come to my bedside to make sure I was all right. I was hooked up to an IV, and when I had to go to the bathroom she helped me out of bed and wheeled the pole for me while I limped across the room, and then she helped me back to bed. The hospital bed had a plastic cover over the mattress, and it made me sweat; I woke up every couple of hours to find the sheets under my back were soaking wet, but she would dry me off.

The next morning, Dr. Youman came in to give me the initial results of the pathology reports and blood work. I was still clinging to my notion that somehow the cancer might not be as bad as we'd thought, until Dr. Youman began to tick off the numbers. He said it appeared from the biopsy and the blood tests that the cancer was spreading rapidly. It was typical of testicular cancer to move up the blood line into the lymph glands, and they had discovered some in my abdomen.

In the 24 hours since I'd first been diagnosed, I'd done as much homework as I could. I knew oncologists broke testicular cancer down into three stages: in stage one, the cancer was confined to the testicles and patients had excellent prognoses; in stage two, the cancer had moved into the abdominal lymph nodes; and in stage three, it had spread to vital organs, such as the lungs. The tests showed that I was stage three, with three different cancers in my body, the most malignant of which was choriocarcinoma, a very aggressive, blood-borne type that was difficult to arrest.

My chemo treatments would begin in a week, via a Grosjean catheter implanted in my chest, and they would last for three months. I would require so many blood tests and intravenous drugs that it was impractical to use standard individual IV needles, so the Grosjean catheter was unavoidable. It was frightening to look at, bulging under my skin, and the opening in my chest seemed unnatural, almost like a gill.

There was another piece of business to discuss: I would be at least temporarily sterile. My first round of chemotherapy was scheduled for the following week, and Youman advised me to bank as much sperm as possible before then. It was the first time the subject of sterility had come up, and I was taken aback. Youman explained that some chemotherapy patients recovered their virility, and some did not; studies showed about a 50-percent return to normalcy after a year. There was a sperm bank two hours away in San Antonio, and Youman recommended I go there.

That night, before we came home from the hospital, my mother went by the oncology unit and picked up all the supplies for my catheter, and my prescriptions for anti-nausea medications, and more literature on testicular cancer. If you've never been to an oncology unit, let me tell you—it can be unsettling. She saw people wrapped in blankets, with no hair, hooked up every which way to IVs, looking pale and deathly sick. My mother gazed around the unit as she waited for the supplies. When they came, she piled it all into a large canvas bag that became our traveling cancer kit, and made her way back to my room. She said, "Son, I just want to let you know that when you go for your treatment, it's not a pleasant sight. But I want you to keep one thing in mind. They're all there for the same reason you are: to get well."

And then she took me home.

ON SATURDAY MORNING I ROSE EARLY AND WENT INTO the bathroom and looked in the mirror—and I stifled a scream. My catheter had a huge blood clot in it and my chest was swollen and caked with blood. I went back into the bedroom and showed Lisa, who stared at it, mute with horror. I yelled for my mother. "Mom, could you come in here!" I said. My mother came racing into my room and examined the catheter. She didn't panic; she just got a washcloth and calmly cleaned it out, and called the hospital. A nurse explained to her that it wasn't uncommon for catheters to clot, and went through a procedure with her for how to prevent it from being infected. But it still looked awful.

My mother hung up and ran to the store, and when she came back she had a box of Band-Aids that glowed in the dark. She put one on the catheter, and that got Lisa and me to laugh. Next, she reached Dr. Youman on the phone. She said, "This catheter is not looking good. I've tried to clean it as much as I can, but maybe we should have it taken out."

Dr. Youman said, "Well, don't do anything yet, because I've decided Lance needs to move up his first chemotherapy treatment. He starts Monday at one o'clock."

"Why?" my mother asked.

I took the phone. Dr. Youman explained that more results had come in from the pathology reports and blood work, and they were worrisome. In a mere 24 hours, the cancer had progressed. Oncologists use something called blood markers to track the progress of the disease: the levels of various proteins in your blood such as human chorionic gonadotropin (HCG) and alpha-fetoprotein (AFP) indicate how much cancer is in the body. My blood counts had risen, in a day.

The cancer was not just spreading, it was galloping, and Youman no longer thought I could afford to wait a week for chemo. I should begin treatment directly, because if the cancer was moving that quickly, every day might count.

I hung up the phone, dispirited. But there was no time to brood; I would have one chance and one chance only to go to the sperm bank in San Antonio: that very afternoon. "This is pathetic," I said to my mother, disgustedly.

The ride to San Antonio was grim. The only thing that relieved the tension was that Kevin Livingston had come home, and he made the trip with me for moral support. I was glad to see him; he has an open face and vivid blue eyes under his cropped black hair, and he always looks like he's on the verge of laughing. It was hard to be in a bad mood around him. We got more help, too: a young man named Cord Shiflet, the son of my architect and friend David Shiflet, offered to drive us.

I sat in the back seat silently as the miles went by, with one nervous thought after another running through my mind. I would have only one chance to bank. I might not be able to have children. I was going to have my first chemo treatment. Would it make me sick?

Finally we arrived at the medical office in San Antonio. Cord and Kevin sat with my mother in the waiting area while a staff nurse escorted me into a private room, and Kevin managed to crack a bad joke, trying to break the terrible mood. "Hey, Lance, you need a magazine?" he said. I grinned, weakly.

I was shown into a room with a lounge chair, a sort of recliner. The lighting was dim, an attempt at ambiance, I guessed. On a small table there was a stack of, yes, magazines. Porn, I saw, disgusted. I hobbled over to the chair, and sighed heavily, and nearly cried. I was in severe pain; the cut from the surgery was right at the top of my groin and met my abdomen. I was depressed and falling apart emotionally from the shock of the diagnosis, and now I was supposed to summon an erection? There was no way. As I lay in the chair, I thought, *This isn't the way it was supposed to happen.* Conceiving a child was supposed to be wreathed in hope, not this sad, solitary, desperate procedure.

I wanted to be a father—quite badly—but I had always assumed it would happen when I was in love. In my early 20s, I'd gone through romantic relationships one after the other. I'd date a woman for a while, and then burn out after just a few months, and stray, and break it off. I dated a girl I'd gone to high school with, I dated a model from Holland, but I was never in a relationship for more than a year. My teammates teasingly named me FedEx for the speed with which I changed girlfriends. The FedEx slogan was "When you absolutely, positively have to have it—overnight." I wasn't married, I had no ties, and it wasn't the deepest period of my life. With Lisa Shiels, though, things were different. By the time I was diagnosed we were very close. She was a bright and serious-minded young woman who was absorbed in her classes at Texas, and the idea of marriage and kids with her had certainly occurred to me. I wasn't sure we were right for each other long-term, but I knew I wanted to be a husband, and I knew, too, that I wanted to be a better father than the ones I had encountered.

I had no choice; I closed my eyes and I did what I had to do.

Out in the waiting room, my mother and my two friends sat, silently. I learned later that while they were sitting there, my mother suddenly turned to Cord and Kevin and said to them, almost angrily, "Now, you boys listen to me. When he comes out, I don't want to hear one word from you. Not one word!" She knew. Somehow, she knew that this was one of the most distressing and utterly cheerless experiences of my life.

When it was over, I came out and handed the vial to a doctor. Cord and Kevin were quiet. I filled out some papers, hastily, and told the

nurses I would send the rest of the information in later. I just wanted
to get out of there. But as we were leaving, the doctor came back out.

"It's a very low count," he said.

The doctor explained that my sperm count was only about a third
of what it should have been; it seemed the cancer had already affected my reproductive capacity. Now the chemo would take its toll,
too.

The drive on the way back was even grimmer than on the way
down. I don't even remember if we ate. I talked to Kevin and Cord
about the magazines. "Can you believe they give you that stuff to look
at?" I said. Kevin and Cord were great; they acted like it was no big
deal, nothing to be embarrassed about, just a very sensible errand,
something that had to be done. I was appreciative, and I took my cue
from them; it was the last time I was self-conscious about the nature
of my illness.

I SPENT THE REST OF THE WEEKEND ON THE COUCH RE-
covering from the surgery. The anesthesia made me woozy, and the incision was excruciating. I rested and watched football while my mother
cooked for me, and we both read up on cancer, exhaustively. "No
stone unturned," my mother said. In between our reading sessions, we
talked about what to do. "How are we going to get rid of this stuff?"
I asked her. We acted as if we could somehow formulate a plan to beat
it, like we had trained in the old days.

That first week my mother picked up all of my prescriptions, col-
lated my medical records, scoured bookstores for cancer material, and
organized my schedule. She bought me a journal to keep notes in and
a visitors' book to keep track of who came to see me. She would
schedule my friends in staggered fashion, so that I would never feel too
alone. We called it the "community calendar," and I had revolving vis-

its, never too many at one time, but never so few as to leave me time to get low, either.

She drew up a three-month calendar to keep track of my chemotherapy treatments, and made lists of my medications and at what time I should take each one. She ran my illness as if it was a project and she was the project manager. She had colored pencils, charts, and time-lines. To her, organization and knowledge would facilitate a cure.

She made an appointment with a nutritionist. I limped off the couch and we drove over, and the nutritionist gave us a guideline for fighting cancer and a list of foods compatible with the chemotherapy drugs: a lot of free-range chicken, broccoli, no cheeses or other fats, and a lot of vitamin C to help combat the toxins of chemo. Immediately, my mother began steaming huge bowls of broccoli for me.

But beneath all of the manic activity, I could tell that my mother was struggling. When she talked to other members of our family on the phone, I could hear a tremor in her voice, and finally she quit calling them when I was around. She tried not to show me all that she felt, but I knew that at night she would go into her room and cry.

On Monday morning, it was time to go public. I held a news conference to announce that I was ill and would not be cycling. Everyone was there, Bill, Lisa, my mother, and several sponsors, and there was a conference call for reporters from Europe as well. Also on the phone were representatives from Cofidis, the French team I was supposed to join in the upcoming season. The room was filled with cameras, and I had to deliver a prepared speech. There was an audible murmur when I said the word "cancer," and I could see the shock and the disbelief on the faces of the reporters and cameramen. A gentleman from Cofidis chimed in on the phone: they pledged their total support in helping me get through the illness and back on the bike.

"I'm determined to fight this disease," I concluded. "And I will win."

———

THAT AFTERNOON, I WALKED INTO YET ANOTHER NON-descript brown brick medical building for my first chemotherapy treatment. I was taken aback by how informal it was: a simple waiting room with some recliners and La-Z-Boys and assorted chairs, a coffee table, and a TV. It looked like somebody's living room full of guests. It might have been a party, except for the giveaway—everybody was attached to his or her very own IV drip.

Dr. Youman explained that the standard treatment protocol for testicular cancer was called BEP, a cocktail of three different drugs, bleomycin, etoposide, and cisplatin, and they were so toxic that the nurses wore radioactive protection when handling them. The most important ingredient of the three was cisplatin, which is actually platinum, and its use against testicular cancer had been pioneered by a man named Dr. Lawrence Einhorn, who practiced at the Indiana University medical center in Indianapolis. Prior to Einhorn's discovery, testicular cancer was almost always fatal—25 years earlier it had killed a Chicago Bears football star named Brian Piccolo, among many others. But the first man who Einhorn had treated with platinum, an Indianapolis schoolteacher, was still alive.

Had I lived 20 years ago, I would have been dead in six months, Youman explained. Most people think Piccolo died of lung cancer, but it started as testicular cancer, and they couldn't save him. He died in 1970 at the age of 26. Since then, cisplatin has become the magic bullet for testicular cancer, and Einhorn's first patient, the Indianapolis teacher, has been cancer-free for over two decades—on his anniversaries they have a big party at his house, and Dr. Einhorn and all his former nurses come to visit him.

I thought, *Bring it on, give me platinum.* But Youman warned that the treatment could make me feel very sick. The three different anti-cancer toxins would be leaked into my system for five hours at a time, over five straight days. They would have a cumulative effect. Anti-emetics would be given to me along with the toxins, to prevent me from suffering severe nausea, but they couldn't curb it entirely.

Chemo is so potent that you can't take it every day. Instead it's administered in three-week cycles; I would take the treatment for one week, and then have two weeks off to allow my body to recover and produce new red blood cells.

Dr. Youman explained everything carefully, preparing us for what we were about to face. When he finished, I had just one question. It was a question I would ask repeatedly over the next several weeks. "What's the cure rate for this?" I asked. "What are my chances?"

Dr. Youman said, "Sixty to sixty-five percent."

My first chemo treatment was strangely undramatic. For one thing, I didn't feel sick. I walked in and chose a chair in the corner, the last one along a wall in a row of six or seven people. My mother kissed me and went off to do some errands, and left me with my fellow patients. I took my place among them.

She had prepared me to be disturbed by my first encounter with other cancer patients, but I wasn't. Instead, I felt a sense of belonging. I was relieved to be able to talk to other people who shared the illness, and compare experiences. By the time my mother got back, I was chatting cheerfully with the guy next to me. He was about my grandfather's age, but we hit it off, and we were jabbering away when my mother walked in. "Hey, Mom," I said brightly. "This is Paul, and he's got prostate cancer."

I HAD TO KEEP MOVING, I TOLD MYSELF. EVERY MORN-ing during that first week of chemo I rose early, put on a pair of sweats and my headphones, and walked. I would stride up the road for an hour or more, breathing and working up a sweat. Every evening, I rode my bike.

Bart Knaggs returned from Orlando with a Mickey Mouse hat he had picked up at Disney World. He handed it to me and told me he knew I would need something to wear when I lost my hair.

We would go riding together, and Kevin Livingston often joined us. Bart made huge maps for us, as large as six feet in diameter. He would get maps of counties from the Department of Highways and cut and paste them together, and we would stand over them choosing new routes for ourselves, long winding rides out in the middle of nowhere. The deal was to always find a new road, someplace we hadn't been before, instead of the same old out-and-back. I couldn't stand to ride the same road twice. The training can be so monotonous that you need newness, even if half the time you end up on a bad piece of road, or get lost. It's okay to get lost sometimes.

Why did I ride when I had cancer? Cycling is so hard, the suffering is so intense, that it's absolutely cleansing. You can go out there with the weight of the world on your shoulders, and after a six-hour ride at a high pain threshold, you feel at peace. The pain is so deep and strong that a curtain descends over your brain. At least for a while you have a kind of hall pass, and don't have to brood on your problems; you can shut everything else out, because the effort and subsequent fatigue are absolute.

There is an unthinking simplicity in something so hard, which is why there's probably some truth to the idea that all world-class athletes are actually running away from something. Once, someone asked me what pleasure I took in riding for so long. "Pleasure?" I said. "I don't understand the question." I didn't do it for pleasure. I did it for pain.

Before the cancer, I had never examined the psychology of jumping on a bicycle and riding for six hours. The reasons weren't especially tangible to me; a lot of what we do doesn't make sense to us while we're doing it. I didn't want to dissect it, because that might let the genie out of the bottle.

But now I knew exactly why I was riding: if I could continue to pedal a bike, somehow I wouldn't be so sick.

The physical pain of cancer didn't bother me so much, because I was used to it. In fact, if I didn't suffer, I'd feel cheated. The more I thought about it, the more cancer began to seem like a race to me. Only the destination had changed. They shared grueling physical aspects, as well as a dependence on time, and progress reports every interval, with checkpoints and a slavish reliance on numbers and blood tests. The only difference was that I had to focus better and harder than I ever did on the bike. With this illness, I couldn't afford impatience or a lapse in concentration; I had to think about living, just making it through, every single moment. The idea was oddly restorative: winning my life back would be the biggest victory.

I was so focused on getting better that during that first round of chemotherapy, I didn't feel anything. Nothing. I even said to Dr. Youman, "Maybe you need to give me more." I didn't realize that I was extremely lucky in how my body tolerated the chemo. Before it was over I would meet other patients who had uncontrollable vomiting after the first cycle, and by the end of my own treatments I would experience a nausea that no drug could get a grip on.

The only thing that suffered at first was my appetite. When you undergo chemotherapy, things taste different because of the chemicals in your body. My mother would fix me a plate of food, and she'd say, "Son, if you're not hungry and you don't want to eat this, it won't hurt my feelings." But I tried to eat. When I woke up from a nap, she would put a plate of sliced fruit and a large bottle of water in front of me. I needed to eat so I could keep moving.

Move, I told myself. I would get up, throw on my warmup clothes, put my Walkman on, and walk. I don't even know how far. I'd walk up the steep hill and out of the front gates, and trudge on up the road.

As long as I could move, I was healthy.

A COUPLE OF DAYS AFTER I STARTED CHEMO, WE OPENED a notification letter from the hospital: *Our records show that you have no health insurance.*

I stared at the letter, uncomprehending. That wasn't possible. I had a health plan with Motorola, and I should have been fully covered. Irritated, I picked up the phone and called Bill Stapleton to read him the letter. Bill calmed me down, and told me he would check into it.

A few hours later, Bill called back. It was a lousy piece of timing, he said. I was in the midst of changing employers, and although my contract with Cofidis had taken effect, the cancer was a preexisting medical condition, for which I was not covered by the Cofidis group plan. My insurance with Motorola had expired. I would have to pay for hospitalizations and the treatments myself, unless Bill could figure something out.

I had cancer, and I had no health insurance.

A lot of terrible realizations hit me one after another in those first few days, and this was only a material matter. Still, it was potentially ruinous. I looked around my house, and started thinking about what to sell. I was wiped out financially, I assumed. I had just gone from making $2 million a year, to nothing. I had some disability insurance, but that was about it. I would have no income, because the companies that sponsored me or paid me would cut me off, surely, since I couldn't race. The Porsche that I so treasured now seemed like an item of pure decadent self-indulgence. I would need every penny to pay the medical bills. I started planning the fire sale. I'd get rid of the Porsche, and some art, and a few other toys.

Within days, the Porsche was gone. I did it for two reasons, first and foremost because I thought I might need every dime for my treatment, and I'd have to live on what was left for the rest of my life. But I think, too, that I was beginning to need to simplify things.

I BECAME A STUDENT OF CANCER. I WENT TO THE biggest bookstore in Austin and bought everything there on the subject. I came home with ten different volumes: diet books, books on coping emotionally, meditation guides. I was willing to consider any option, no matter how goofy. I read about flaxseed oil, which was supposed to be "a true aid" against arthritis, heart infarction, cancer, and other diseases. I read about soy powder, a "proven anti-cancer fighter." I read *Yoga Journal,* and became deeply if only momentarily interested in something called The Raj, "an invitation to perfect health." I tore out pages of *Discover* magazine, and collected newspaper stories on far-off clinics and far-fetched cures. I perused a pamphlet about the Clinic of the Americas in the Dominican Republic, describing "an absolutely certain cure for cancer."

I devoured what Bart had given me, and every time he called, I said, "What else you got?" I had never been a devoted reader, but now I became voracious. Bart went to Amazon.com and cleaned them out on the subject. "Look, do you want me to feed you what I find?" he asked.

"Yeah, I want everything. Everything, everything."

Here I was, a high-school graduate who'd received an eclectic education in Europe, and now I was reading medical journals. I had always liked to study financial magazines and architectural-design magazines, but I didn't care much for books; I had an impossibly short attention span and I couldn't sit still for that long. Now all of a sudden I had to tackle blood counts and basic oncology. It was a second education, and there were days that I thought, *Well, I might as well go back to school and try to become a doctor, because I'm becoming so well-versed in this.*

I sat on the sofa flipping through books, talking on the phone, reading off numbers. I wanted to know exactly what my odds were, so I could figure out how to beat them. The more research I did, the better I felt my chances were—even though what I was reading suggested that they weren't very good. But knowledge was more reassuring than ignorance: at least I knew what I was dealing with, or thought I did anyway.

There was an odd commonality in the language of cancer and the language of cycling. They were both about blood. In cycling, one way of cheating is to take a drug that boosts your red bloodcell count. In fighting cancer, if my hemoglobin fell below a certain level, the doctors would give me the very same drug, Epogen. There was a baseline of numbers I had to meet in my blood tests, and the doctors measured my blood for the very same thing they measured in cycling: my threshold for physiological stress.

I mastered a whole new language, terms like ifosfamide (a chemotherapy drug), seminoma (a kind of tumor), and lactate dehydrogenase (LDH, another blood marker). I began to throw around phrases like "treatment protocol." I wanted to know it all. I wanted second, third, and fourth opinions.

I began to receive mountains of mail, get-well cards, best wishes, and off-the-wall suggestions for cures, and I read them all. Reading the mail was a way to keep from brooding, so in the evenings Lisa and my mother and I would sort through the letters, and answer as many as possible.

One evening, I opened a letter with an embossed letterhead from Vanderbilt University's medical center. The writer was a man named Dr. Steven Wolff, the head of the bone-marrow transplant department. In the letter, Dr. Wolff explained that he was a professor of medicine and an oncologist, as well as an ardent cycling fan, and he wanted to help in any way he could. He urged me to explore all the various treatment options, and offered to be available for any advice or support. Two things about the letter drew my attention; the first was Wolff's obvious cycling knowledge, and the other was a paragraph that urged me in strong terms to get a second opinion from Dr. Larry Einhorn himself at Indiana University because he was the foremost expert on the disease. Wolff added, "You should note that there are equally effective chemotherapy treatments that could minimize possible side effects to not compromise your racing capabilities."

I picked up the phone and dialed Wolff. "Hi, this is Lance Armstrong," I said. Wolff was taken aback, but he recovered quickly, and after we exchanged a few pleasantries, he began a hesitant inquiry about my treatment. Wolff explained that he was reluctant to encroach on the authority of my doctors in Austin, but he wanted to help. I told him that I was on the standard treatment protocol for testicular cancer with lung metastasis, BEP.

"My prognosis isn't good," I said.

From that moment on, my treatment became a medical collaboration. Previously, I thought of medicine as something practiced by individual doctors on individual patients. The doctor was all-knowing and all-powerful, the patient was helpless. But it was beginning to dawn on me that there was nothing wrong with seeking a cure from a combination of people and sources, and that the patient was as important as the doctor. Dr. Reeves was my urologist, Dr. Youman my oncologist, and now Dr. Wolff became my friend and treatment advocate, a third medical eye and someone to whom I could turn to ask questions. Each doctor involved played a crucial role. No one person could take sole responsibility for the state of my health, and most important, I began to share the responsibility with them.

"What's your HCG level?" Wolff asked me.

HCG is the endocrine protein that stimulates women's ovaries, I had learned, and it was a telling blood marker because it should not be present in healthy males. I shuffled through the papers, looking at the various figures. "It says a hundred and nine," I said.

"Well, that's high," Wolff said. "But not extraordinary."

As I stared at the page, I saw another notation after the number.

"Uh, what's this 'K' mean?" I asked.

He was silent for a moment, and so was I.

"It means it's a hundred and nine thousand," Wolff said.

If a count of 109 was high, then what was *109,000?* Wolff began to ask me about my other marker levels, AFB and LDH. I shot questions back at him. "What does this mean?" I asked bluntly.

Wolff explained that there was too much HCG in my body, even with the lung tumors. Where was it coming from? He gently suggested that perhaps I should explore other therapies, more aggressive treatment. Then he let me have it: the HCG level automatically put me in the worst prognosis category.

Something else bothered Wolff. Bleomycin was extremely toxic on the liver and lungs, he explained. In his view, treatment was very personal; what might be right for one patient wasn't necessarily right for another, and for my case, bleomycin might be the wrong choice. A cyclist needs his lung capacity the way he needs his legs, and prolonged exposure to bleomycin would almost certainly end my career. There were other drugs, Wolffe suggested. I had choices.

"There are some guys who are the world's best at treating this," Wolff said. He told me he was a friend of Einhorn and the other oncologists at the Indiana University medical center in Indianapolis. He also recommended two other cancer centers—one in Houston and one in New York. Moreover, he offered to arrange consultations for me. Immensely relieved, I accepted.

Once again, my mother leaped into action. By the next morning, she had gathered all of my medical records and faxed them to Houston and Indianapolis for the consults. I was out riding my bike at about 10 A.M. when a reply came from the Houston facility. Two doctors were on a conference call, both oncologists. My mother listened to two disembodied voices as they discussed my case with her.

"We've reviewed the information," one said. "Why haven't you had an MRI done on the brain?"

"Well, why would we need that?" my mother asked.

"His numbers are so high that we believe he has it in his brain, too," he said.

"You gotta be kidding me," my mother said.

"Normally when we see numbers like that, it's because it's in the brain. We feel he needs more aggressive treatment."

Stunned, my mother said, "But he just started chemotherapy."

"Look," one of them said. "We don't think your son is going to make it at this rate."

"Don't do this, okay?" she said. "I have fought for this child my entire life."

"We feel you should come down here immediately, and start treatments with us."

"Lance will be back in a little while," my mother said, shakily. "I'll talk to him, and we'll call you back."

A few minutes later, I walked in the door, and my mother said, "Son, I've got to talk to you." I could see that she was a wreck, and I had that familiar sinking sensation in my stomach. As my mother tremulously summarized what the doctors had said, I didn't respond, I just sat there silently—it seemed like the more serious matters grew, the quieter I became. After a minute, I calmly told her that I wanted to talk to the doctors myself, and hear what they had to say.

I called them back, and I listened as they reiterated what they had already told my mother. Wearily, I told them that I wanted to go to Houston and see them as soon as possible. After I got off the phone, I paged Dr. Youman. I gave him a brief encapsulation of my conversation with the Houston doctors. "Dr. Youman, they think I have it in my brain. They say I should have a brain MRI."

"Well, I was going to have you in for one tomorrow," Youman said. "You're actually already scheduled for noon."

Dr. Youman told me that he had scheduled the MRI because he had been thinking along the same lines, that it had probably moved into my brain.

I called Steve Wolff, and told him about the conversation. I said that I intended to go to Houston the next day. Steve agreed that I should go, but he again recommended that I also talk to the people at Indiana University, because it was the epicenter for dealing with testicular cancer. Everyone took their treatments from the protocols established by Einhorn, so why didn't I go straight to the source? Steve told me that Einhorn was traveling in Australia, but he offered to refer me to Einhorn's chief associate, Dr. Craig Nichols. I agreed, and he called Nichols to ask for a consultation on my behalf.

The next morning, I reported to the hospital for the MRI. For moral support, Lisa, my mother, and Bill Stapleton all came with me, and my grandmother flew in from Dallas as well. As soon as I saw Dr. Youman, I said fatalistically, "I fully expect that I have it in my brain. I already know that's what you're going to tell me."

A brain MRI is a claustrophobic procedure in which you are passed through a tunnel so tight that it practically touches your nose and forehead and makes you feel that you might suffocate. I hated it.

The results of the scan came back almost immediately. My mother and grandmother and Bill waited in the lobby, but I wanted Lisa with me in Dr. Youman's office. I gripped her hand. Dr. Youman took one look at the image and said, reluctantly, "You have two spots on your brain."

Lisa covered her eyes. I was braced for it, but she wasn't. Neither was my mother, who sat in the lobby waiting for me. I walked outside, and I simply said, "We need to go to Houston." That was all I had to say; she knew the rest.

Dr. Youman said, "Okay, why don't you go to talk to the Houston people. That's a very good idea." I already knew he was an excellent doctor, but now I appreciated his lack of ego. He would remain my local oncologist, and I would see him for countless more blood tests and checkups, but thanks to his generous spirit and willingness to collaborate with others in my treatment, he also became my friend.

Lisa and my mother could not keep from crying; they sat in the lobby with tears running from their eyes. But I was oddly unemotional. It had been a busy week, I thought to myself. I was diagnosed on a Wednesday, had surgery Thursday, was released Friday night, banked sperm on Saturday, had a press conference announcing to the world that I had testicular cancer on Monday morning, started chemo on Monday afternoon. Now it was Thursday, and it was in my brain. This opponent was turning out to be much tougher than I'd thought. I couldn't seem to get any *good* news: *It's in your lungs, it's stage three, you have no insurance, now it's in your brain.*

We drove home, and my mother composed herself and sat at the fax machine feeding more papers into it for the doctors in Houston. Lisa sat in the living room, seeming lost. I called Bart, and told him about my plans. Bart asked if I wanted company on the trip, and I said yes. We would leave at 6 A.M. the next day.

But believe it or not, there was a certain relief in hearing the worst news yet—because I felt like that was the end of it all. No doctor could tell me anything more; now I knew every terrible thing in the world.

Each time I was more fully diagnosed, I asked my doctors hard questions. *What are my chances?* I wanted to know the numbers. My percentage was shrinking daily. Dr. Reeves told me 50 percent, "but really I was thinking twenty," he admitted to me later. If he was perfectly honest, he would have told me that he nearly wept when he examined me, because he thought he was looking at a terminally ill 25-year-old, and he couldn't help but think of his own son, who was my age. If Bart Knaggs had been totally candid, he would have told me that when his prospective father-in-law, who was a doctor, had heard that the cancer had moved into my lungs, he said to Bart, "Well, your friend is dead."

What are my chances? It was a question I would repeat over and over. But it was irrelevant, wasn't it? It didn't matter, because the medical odds don't take into account the unfathomable. There is no proper way to estimate somebody's chances, and we shouldn't try, because we can never be entirely right, and it deprives people of hope. Hope that is the only antidote to fear.

Those questions, *Why me? What are my chances?* were unknowable, and I would even come to feel that they were too self-absorbed. For most of my life I had operated under a simple schematic of winning and losing, but cancer was teaching me a tolerance for ambiguities. I was coming to understand that the disease doesn't discriminate or listen to the odds—it will decimate a strong person with a wonderful attitude, while it somehow miraculously spares the weaker person who is resigned to failure. I had always assumed that if I won bike races, it made me a stronger and more worthy person. Not so.

Why me? Why anybody? I was no more or less valuable than the man sitting next to me in the chemo center. It was not a question of worthiness.

What is stronger, fear or hope? It's an interesting question, and perhaps even an important one. Initially, I was very fearful and without much hope, but as I sat there and absorbed the full extent of my illness, I refused to let the fear completely blot out my optimism. Something told me that fear should never fully rule the heart, and I decided not to be afraid.

I wanted to live, but whether I would or not was a mystery, and in the midst of confronting that fact, even at that moment, I was beginning to sense that to stare into the heart of such a fearful mystery wasn't a bad thing. To be afraid is a priceless education. Once you have been that scared, you know more about your frailty than most people, and I think that changes a man. I was brought low, and there was nothing to take refuge in but the philosophical: this disease would force me to ask more of myself as person than I ever had before, and to seek out a different ethic.

A couple of days earlier, I had received an e-mail from a military guy stationed in Asia. He was a fellow cancer patient, and he wanted to tell me something. "You don't know it yet," he wrote, "but we're the lucky ones."

I'd said aloud, "This guy's a nut."

What on earth could he mean?

five

CONVERSATIONS WITH CANCER

There was a disquieting intimacy to the idea that something uninvited was living in my head. When something climbs straight into your mind, that's way personal. I decided to get personal right back, and I began to talk to it, engaging in an inner conversation with cancer. I tried to be firm in my discussions. "You picked the wrong guy," I told it. "When you looked around for a body to try to live in, you made a big mistake when you chose mine."

But even as I said the words, I knew they were just competitive braggadocio. The face that looked back at me from the mirror that morning was pale and bleary-eyed, and my mouth was stretched into a thin hard line. In the sound of my own inner voice I heard an unfamiliar note: uncertainty.

I tried negotiating with it. *If the deal is that I never cycle again, but I get to live, I'll take it,* I thought. *Show me the dotted line, and I'll sign. I'll do something else, I'll go back to school, I'll be a trash man, do anything. Just let me live.*

We left before sunrise for the drive to Houston. My mother was at the wheel of her Volvo and I rode with Lisa in the backseat, which was unlike me. I never turned the driving over to anyone else—that right there tells you how preoccupied I was. We were virtually wordless for the three-hour trip, exhausted and lost in our own thoughts; none of us had been able to sleep well the previous night. My mother pushed the accelerator, as if she just wanted to get it over with. She was so distracted, she almost hit a dog.

Houston is a gigantic metroplex of a city, with traffic jams choking the freeways. Just driving through it was nerve-racking. We finally found the hospital at 9 A.M., and filed into the lobby waiting area, and that's exactly what we did—waited, for the next two hours. We were too early. Sitting in the lobby, I felt like we were in another traffic jam.

It was a sprawling university hospital and teaching facility, with huge, echoing hallways teeming with people—sick people, crying babies, worried family members, brusque hospital administrators, harried nurses, doctors, interns. The fluorescent tubes in the ceiling shed a white, leaky sodium light so typical of hospitals, an unrelenting flat beam that makes even the healthy people look pale and tense. It seemed like we waited forever, and as I sat there, I grew increasingly agitated. I flipped through magazines and drummed a pencil on the arm of the chair, and made calls on my cell phone.

Finally, the doctor I had spoken to appeared and we met face-to-face: he was the picture of a smart young oncologist, a well-groomed man with clipped manners and the lean physique of a runner beneath his lab coat.

"I've been following you," he said. "I'm glad you're here."

But once the pleasantries were over, he had a bedside manner that was terse and cold. As soon as we sat down, he began to outline a treatment protocol. He would continue treating me with bleomycin, he said, but his regimen would be much more caustic than what Youman had prescribed.

"You will crawl out of here," he said.

My eyes widened, and so did my mother's. I was taken aback. He continued. "I'm going to kill you," he said. "Every day, I'm going to kill you, and then I'm going to bring you back to life. We're going to hit you with chemo, and then hit you again, and hit you again. You're not going to be able to walk." He said it point-blank. "We're practically going to have to teach you how to walk again, after we're done."

Because the treatment would leave me infertile, I would probably never have kids. Because the bleomycin would tear up my lungs, I would never be able to race a bike again. I would suffer immense pain. The more he talked, the more I recoiled at the vivid images of my enfeeblement. I asked him why the treatment had to be so harsh. "You're worst-case," he said. "But I feel this is your only shot, at this hospital."

By the time he finished, my mother was trembling, and Lisa looked shell-shocked. Bart was angry. He interrupted and tried to ask a couple of questions about alternative treatments. Bart is a real questioner and note-taker, a very thorough man, and he was worried and protective. The doctor cut him off.

"Look, your chances aren't great," he said to me. "But they're a lot better if you come here than they are if you go anywhere else."

I asked him what his thoughts were about Dr. Einhorn's protocol in Indianapolis. He was dismissive. "You can go to Indiana, but chances are you'll be back here. Their therapy won't work for an advanced case like yours."

Finally, he concluded his presentation. He wanted me to start chemotherapy with him immediately. "This is the only place to get this sort of treatment, and if you don't do it, I can't promise you what will happen," he said.

I told him I wanted to think about what he had said over lunch, and I would come back in the afternoon with an answer.

We drove around Houston in a daze. Finally we found a sandwich shop, but none of us felt much like eating after hearing such a dire summation of my case. I felt pressure to make a quick decision: it was Friday, and he wanted me to begin treatment Monday.

I was discouraged. I could accept the idea that I was perilously sick, but the idea of being reduced to feebleness was the most depressing thought of all. Listlessly, I went over the pros and cons of what he had said, and asked for feedback from my mother and Lisa and Bart. How do you discuss such a matter? I tried to put a positive spin on the consultation, and set forth the opinion that maybe this doctor's competitiveness and self-confidence were good. But I could see that my mother had plainly been terrified by him.

The protocol sounded so much more severe than what I would receive anywhere else. *I won't walk, I won't have children, I won't ride,* I thought. Ordinarily, I was the sort who went in for overkill: aggressive training, aggressive racing. But for once I thought, *Maybe this is too much. Maybe this is more than I need.*

I decided to call Dr. Wolff to ask his opinion. The more I talked to him, the better I liked him; he was all gray matter and good sense, with no ego. I outlined the proposed protocol and the repercussions. "He wants me to start treatment right away, and he's expecting an answer this afternoon."

Wolff was quiet on his end of the phone. I could hear him thinking. "It wouldn't hurt you to get one more opinion," he said finally. Wolff didn't think I needed to make a decision that day, and he suggested that I at least visit the Indiana medical center. The more I thought about it, the more it seemed like a good recommendation. Why not go to Indianapolis and see the people who wrote the book on testicular cancer, the protocol that all the other doctors used?

On the car phone, I called Dr. Craig Nichols, Einhorn's associate. I explained that my situation was grave and that I wanted additional opinions and was in a hurry to get them. "Can I come see you now?" I asked.

Nichols replied that he had been expecting my call. "We can see you right away," he said. Could I get there in time to meet early the next morning? It was a Saturday. I learned later that it wasn't completely a case of special treatment; the IU staff does not turn away cases, no matter how bad, and they do phone consultations with patients and other doctors around the world daily.

By now it was three o'clock, and I was apprehensive about going back to the Houston facility to retrieve my medical records. The doctor there was obviously eager to treat me, but he had frightened me, too. When I told him I wanted to wait a day or two to make my decision, he was pleasant, and wished me luck. "Just don't wait too long," he said.

The decision to go to Indianapolis lifted my mother's spirits somewhat, and she took charge. She got on her cell phone to Bill Stapleton's office, and reached his assistant, Stacy Pounds. "Stacy, we need to be on a plane to Indianapolis," she said. Then we piled in the car and raced to the Houston airport. We dumped my mother's Volvo in the long-term parking lot. None of us had any clothes or toothbrushes because we thought we were going to Houston for a day trip. When we got to the ticket counter, we discovered that Stacy had not only managed to get us four seats, but had gotten us upgrades as well.

When we landed in Indianapolis my mother took charge again, and rented us a car. It was cold in Indianapolis, but she discovered that there was a hotel adjoining the hospital with a covered walkway. She checked us in there, and we collapsed in our rooms. It would be another short night, because we were scheduled to meet with Dr. Nichols early the next morning.

I ROSE IN ANOTHER PREDAWN, AND STOOD COMBING my hair in the mirror. I had already cut it close to my head, in anticipation of the effects of chemo. Now a big thatch of it came away in the comb. I put on a cap.

I went down to the lobby. The hotel had a continental breakfast buffet with cereal and fruit in the dining room, and my mother was already there. As I joined her at the table, I took off the cap.

"My hair's falling out," I announced.

My mother tried to smile. "Well, we knew that it would."

I tucked my X rays and other records under my arm, and we walked across the street to the hospital in the chilly darkness.

The IU medical center is a standard teaching hospital housed in a large institutional-looking building. We took the elevator to the oncology offices, where we were ushered into a conference room with a large plate-glass window.

As we walked in, the sun was just beginning to come up, and the room was suffused with color. For much of the next hour the sun continued to rise steadily through the window, shimmering, which may have contributed to the sense of well-being I experienced.

We met the doctors who would consult with me. Craig Nichols was a distinguished-looking man with a cropped beard and an understated air. He carried a cup of coffee in a Styrofoam cup. I wasn't drinking coffee, and I missed it badly. I had given it up because the nutrition books said to; if no caffeine could help save my life, then I didn't intend to drink a drop. But I stared at Nichols's cup, feeling pangs of withdrawal.

"Where do you stand on coffee?" I asked.

"Well, it's probably not the best thing for you," he said, "but a cup here and a cup there probably won't kill you."

Accompanying Nichols was Scott Shapiro, a neurosurgeon. Shapiro was a tall and stoop-shouldered man who looked exactly like the actor Abe Vigoda, with deep-set eyes and bushy eyebrows. Dr. Nichols summed up my case to Shapiro: I was diagnosed with testicular cancer and it had metastasized. "The workup found mets in his chest, and two brain mets," Nichols said to Shapiro.

We sat down, and as we began to talk the sun glowed through the glass. The hospital was very quiet, and Nichols had a calm, plain-spoken manner that contributed to the sense of peacefulness I felt. As he talked, I studied him. He was very relaxed, with a habit of leaning against walls, tilting back in chairs with his hands behind his head, and clearing his throat. But there was clearly a tremendous confidence beneath his mildness. He began to grow on me.

"We, *unh,*" he said, clearing his throat, "feel good about your, *unh,* chances."

I told Nichols we had just come from Houston. I expected him to be as dismissive as his counterpart had been, but instead, he was gracious. He said, "It's a fine facility and we appreciate the work they do." He then took my medical records and began to review them. He stuck my X rays up on the light board, and I stared over his shoulder at them as he pointed out the areas of abnormality in my chest, counting 12 tumors in all—"multiple nodules on both sides," as he put it. Some of them were specks, and some measured as large as 2.7 centimeters. Then he turned to my brain scan and showed me the two areas of abnormality right under the skull. They were grape-sized white spots.

I was very attentive—there is something about staring at your brain metastases that focuses a person. Nichols made suggestions, almost casually, about my prognosis and how he would fight the disease. His presentation was simple and straightforward.

"You're in an advanced stage, and the brain lesions complicate things," he said. He explained that typically brain lesions aren't treated with chemo because of the blood-brain barrier, a kind of physiological moat that guards the brain, blocking the entry of drugs like those used in chemotherapy. The options were radiation and/or surgery. Nichols favored surgery.

As usual, I wanted hard, precise information. *What are my chances?*

"Well, you got a poor start," Nichols said, meaning I had been diagnosed late. "The percentages are unfavorable. But this is potentially curable. I think you have almost a coin-flip of a chance."

Nichols was sober and realistic, but he exuded optimism, too. In testicular cancer, there is almost always a chance of cure now, thanks to the use of platinum, and he had seen people with more advanced disease than I had who survived. "We see all the very hard cases here," he said. "Even though you're in the poor-prognosis category, we've cured a lot worse."

Then Nichols stunned me: he said that he would like to tailor my treatment to get me back on the bike. That was the one thing no doctor besides Steve Wolff had said to me. Not one. I was so taken aback that at first I didn't trust what he was saying. The trip to Houston had so deflated me, particularly the description of the rigors of treatment and the extreme measures it would take to save me. My highest priority was survival. "Just help me live," I said.

But Nichols was not only confident that I could live, he seemed to feel there was a chance I could race again. He wouldn't compromise my chances of living, but he wanted to alter my protocol to preserve my lungs. There was another protocol of platinum-based chemo called VIP (vinblastine, etoposide, ifosfamide, cisplatin), which was a much more caustic regimen in the short term, but which in the long term would not be as debilitating to my lungs as bleomycin. With ifos-famide, he said, I would have more nausea and vomiting and short-term discomfort. If I could withstand three cycles of VIP, in addition to the BEP cycle I had already undergone, I just might get rid of the cancer and be able to recover enough physically to compete.

"You mean we can do that instead of what everyone else is doing?" my mother asked. "No bleomycin?"

"We don't want his lungs to be affected," Nichols said.

Nichols continued: he favored surgery to remove the brain tumors. The standard treatment for brain tumors was radiation, but radiation can have long-term side effects on the central nervous system; some patients who undergo it have intellection deterioration and cognitive and coordination disturbance. "They're not quite the same after radi-ation," he said. In my case one potential effect could be a slight loss of balance. Nothing serious to the ordinary person, but enough to keep me from riding a bike down an Alp—balance is something you need in that situation.

Shapiro took over the discussion. I studied him: in addition to his resemblance to the sad-eyed Vigoda, there was the matter of what he was wearing: an Adidas sweatsuit with the signature stripes down the side and zippers at the bottom, over which he wore the more tradi-tional lab coat. His hair curled over his collar. *This guy is a brain surgeon?* I wondered. He seemed entirely too casual to be a doctor at all.

"Let's look at the MRIs and the CT scans," Shapiro said easily.

Nichols handed them over. Shapiro popped the images up on the X ray board, and as he regarded them, he began to slowly nod.

"Mmmm, yep," he said. "I can handle this. No problem."

"No *problem?*" I said.

Shapiro pointed to the lesions and said that they appeared to be on the surface of my brain, and should therefore be relatively easy to get at, using something called frameless stereotactics, a technology that al-

lowed him to pinpoint precisely where the cancer was and conse-
quently make a relatively small incision.

"It allows us to isolate the lesions before we operate, so that our
time in the cranial area is a fourth of what it would have been before,"
he said.

"What are the risks?" I asked.

"With a young person, the problems of anesthesia are minimal.
There's not much risk of infection or hemorrhage, either, and only a
small risk of seizure. The main risk is that you might come out of it
with some weakness on one side of the body. It's a simple procedure,
and you seem like a pretty strong character. It should be a walk in the
park."

I was tired, and in a state of disbelief. It made me blunt. "You'll have
to convince me you know what you're doing," I said.

"Look, I've done a large number of these," Shapiro said. "I've never
had anyone die, and I've never made anyone worse."

"Yeah, but why should you be the person who operates on my
head?"

"Because as good as you are at cycling"—he paused—"I'm a lot
better at brain surgery."

I laughed, and knew that I liked him. By then it was late morning,
and I rose from my chair and told them that we would think about
what they had said over lunch, and that I would make a decision later
that day.

First, I wanted to have another talk with my friends and my mother.
These were stressful decisions. I had to choose my doctors and my
place of treatment, and it wasn't like choosing a mutual fund, either.
If I invested in a mutual fund, I'd ask, *What's my rate of return over five
years?* But this was entirely different. The rate of return in this instance was a matter of life and death.

We went across the street to a mall, and found a brew pub. Everyone was quiet at lunch. Too quiet. My mother, Lisa, and Bart were afraid of influencing me; they all thought I should make my own decision about where to be treated. I asked them for comments, but couldn't seem to draw them into it.

I kept trying. "Well, you know, they say in Houston there's a good chance I'll be cured, but here they want to change my protocol, and maybe that's good." Nobody replied, or gave the slightest hint of an opinion. They were totally noncommittal. They wanted a decision, but it had to be mine, not theirs.

While I ate, I thought it over. I wanted to be sure I had done a good job of evaluating the doctors and understanding their treatment plans. I was at ground zero, I had conceded my career, but Dr. Nichols and Dr. Shapiro didn't seem to think I had to make that concession yet. I decided I had confidence in them, in their purposely laid-back styles, their lack of ego, and their refusal to be rattled by me. They were exactly who they appeared to be: two wrinkled, tired, yet very learned doctors, and I suspected there were none better.

I had tried to ask some tough questions, but Nichols was imperturbable, and candid. He wasn't going to get suckered into a bidding war, or try to sell his shop over another. He was extremely professional, and secure in his credibility.

Suddenly, I blurted, "Well, these guys really seem like they know what they're doing. And I really like them. I like this place. And if I'm going to have to have surgery, Dr. Shapiro doesn't seem worried at all. So I think I'm gonna come here."

Their faces lit up. "I totally agree," Bart said, finally going out on a limb.

My mother said, "I think you're right."

We returned to the IU medical center, and I met with Dr. Nichols again. "This is where I want to do my treatment," I said.

"Okay, good," Nichols said. "You need to be back here on Monday to take some measurements, and Tuesday we'll operate on the brain."

Nichols said that immediately after the surgery I would start the new chemotherapy regimen with him. He brought in the chief oncology nurse, LaTrice Haney, who would be working with me, and we sat down to map out a treatment schedule.

"You can't kill me," I said. "Hit me with everything you got, just dump it all on me. Whatever you give to other people, give me double. I want to make sure we get it all. Let's kill this damn thing."

Nichols and LaTrice wanted to disabuse me of that notion right away. "Let me assure you, I can kill you," Nichols said. "It's possible." I was under the misperception, in part because of the conversation in Houston, that they had to bombard me to cure me, but chemo is so toxic that too much of it would destroy my system. Nichols actually wanted to wait a week to begin treating me, because my white blood cell count was still low from the first cycle of chemo. Only when I was physically ready would I begin a VIP chemo cycle.

LaTrice Haney took over the conversation. She was a very correct and expert-seeming nurse, although I would discover that she had a sneaky wit. Her fluency on the subject of chemotherapy seemed equal to the doctors' as she guided me through every element of the protocol, explaining not just what each one did, but why it worked, in an almost teacherly way. I tried to take in all of the information—I was determined to stay involved in my health, in the decision-making. My mother was still anxious, of course.

"How sick will he be?" she asked.

"He will probably have episodes of nausea, he may have vomiting," LaTrice said. "But there are new medications out, recent ones that can minimize his vomiting, if not eliminate it."

LaTrice told me that every drop of chemo that went into my body would be carefully counted, as would everything that came out. Her explanations were so calm and succinct that when she was through, I didn't have any questions, and my mother seemed comforted. La Trice had answered everything.

A WEEK LATER, WE RETURNED TO INDIANAPOLIS. My mother carried all my records in her bag, as well as a huge Ziploc full of my vitamins and medicines. By now she had been living out of one small overnight case for almost three weeks, and she didn't even have a sweater. It was cool in Indianapolis, so she borrowed a blanket off the plane to keep warm.

At the IU medical center, we went through another laborious check-in process, with my mother digging in her bag for my records. An administrator took down all of the pertinent information and asked us various questions.

"What kind of food do you like?" she asked.

I said, "I can't have sugars. I can't have beef. I can't have cheese products. And I have to have free-range chicken."

She just stared back at me, and said, "What *can* you eat?"

It was a teaching hospital, not a catering service, I realized. But my mother was furious. She stood up, all 5-foot-3 of her, and said, "We're getting ready to face brain surgery tomorrow, and don't even try this with me. We have a nutritionist who has recommended certain things. If you can't do it, fine. We'll get our own food." From then on, whenever my mother visited the hospital she went shopping for me.

Next, we went to our room, and my mother decided it was too noisy. It was right by the nurses' station, and she thought it would disturb me to hear them talking outside my door, so she insisted that they change my room, and I was moved to the end of the hall, where it was quieter.

That afternoon, I saw Dr. Shapiro for the preliminaries to surgery.

One charming feature of frameless stereotactics entailed placing colored dots all over my skull to mark the locations of the tumors and the places where Shapiro would make his incisions to get to them.

Somehow, those dots made the surgery more immediate. It struck me that they put those dots on my head so that Shapiro would know where to *cut into my skull.* There was no easy way to say it; it was where the surgeon would *crack my head open.*

"LaTrice," I said, "the idea of cutting my head open, I just don't know if I can deal with that."

I met a wall. Much as I wanted to be positive and unafraid, all I knew was, when people get brain tumors, they don't live. The rest I figured was curable; my other organs and appendages weren't as important. But the brain, that was the big one. I remembered a rhyme I'd heard somewhere, "Once you touch the brain you're never the same."

The people around me were as frightened as I was, or more so. It seemed everyone I knew had flown in to be with me: Och, Chris Carmichael, Bill, Kevin. I wanted them around, and I knew they were glad to be there, because it made them feel like they could do something to help. But I could see the fear in their faces, in their widened eyes and their false cheerfulness, so I tried to rally, and to hide my own uncertainty.

"I'm ready to crush this thing," I announced. "I'm ready for this surgery. You won't find me sitting around trembling, scared to let them take me."

One thing you realize when you're sick is that you aren't the only person who needs support—sometimes you have to be the one who supports others. My friends shouldn't always have to be the ones saying: "You're going to make it." Sometimes I had to be the one who reassured them, and said, "I'm going to make it. Don't worry."

We watched the World Series and tried to act like we were interested in the outcome—as much as anybody really cares about baseball before brain surgery. We chatted about the stock market, and about bicycle racing. The e-mails and cards kept pouring in, from people I didn't even know or hadn't heard from in years, and we sat around reading them aloud.

I felt a sudden urgency to assess my financial worth. I explained the health-insurance problem to Och and Chris, and we got paper and pencils and began totaling up my assets. "Let's see where I am," I said. "We've got to get this wired tight. I need to have a plan, so I can feel like I'm controlling this thing." I had enough saved up to go to college, we decided—if I sold my house. I didn't want to sell it, but I tried to be philosophical. Hey, I got dealt a bad hand. If I needed the money, that's what I would have to do. I added up my cash, and how much was in my retirement account.

Lot: $220,000. Pool and landscaping: $60,000. Furniture and art: $300,000. Fixtures: $50,000.

Later in the day, Shapiro came to my room. "We need to discuss the surgery," he said in a serious tone.

"What are you talking about?" I said. "This is relatively minor, right?"

"Well, it's a little more serious than that."

Shapiro said that the tumors were in two tricky spots: one was over my vision field and the other was over a center of coordination. So that explained my blurry vision. He said he would tailor the operation to be precise, keeping the incisions as small as possible, hopefully making them within one millimeter of the lesions. There would be no huge incisions like in the old days. Still, I shuddered at his description of the procedure. I don't think I had fully admitted the severity of the operation to myself; I thought it sounded easy—he would just go in and scrape off the lesions. But now that he went into the details, it hit home that he would be operating in areas where the slightest errors could cost me my eyesight or my movement and motor skills.

Shapiro could see that I was beginning to get truly frightened. "Look, nobody ever *wants* brain surgery," he said. "If you aren't scared, you aren't normal."

Shapiro assured me that I would bounce back from the surgery quickly: I would spend just one day in intensive care and, after another day of recovery, I would get straight down to business with my chemotherapy.

That night, my mother, Bill, Och, Chris, and the rest of the group took me across the street to the mall to get something to eat at a nice continental-cuisine restaurant. I couldn't eat much. I still had the dots on my head from the frameless stereotactics, and a hospital bracelet on my wrist, but I no longer cared how I looked. So what if I had dots on my head? I was just happy to get out of the hospital and move around. People stared, but it didn't matter. Tomorrow, my head would be shaved.

HOW DO YOU CONFRONT YOUR OWN DEATH? SOMEtimes I think the blood-brain barrier is more than just physical, it's emotional, too. Maybe there's a protective mechanism in our psyche that prevents us from accepting our mortality unless we absolutely have to.

The night before brain surgery, I thought about death. I searched out my larger values, and I asked myself, if I was going to die, did I want to do it fighting and clawing or in peaceful surrender? What sort of character did I hope to show? Was I content with myself and what I had done with my life so far? I decided that I was essentially a good person, although I could have been better—but at the same time I understood that the cancer didn't care.

I asked myself what I believed. I had never prayed a lot. I hoped hard, I wished hard, but I didn't pray. I had developed a certain distrust of organized religion growing up, but I felt I had the capacity to be a spiritual person, and to hold some fervent beliefs. Quite simply, I believed I had a responsibility to be a good person, and that meant fair, honest, hardworking, and honorable. If I did that, if I was good to my family, true to my friends, if I gave back to my community or to some cause, if I wasn't a liar, a cheat, or a thief, then I believed that should be enough. At the end of the day, if there was indeed some Body or presence standing there to judge me, I hoped I would be judged on whether I had lived a true life, not on whether I believed in a certain book, or whether I'd been baptized. If there was indeed a God at the end of my days, I hoped he didn't say, "But you were never a Christian, so you're going the other way from heaven." If so, I was going to reply, "You know what? You're right. Fine."

I believed, too, in the doctors and the medicine and the surgeries— I believed in that. I believed in them. A person like Dr. Einhorn, that's someone to believe in, I thought, a person with the mind to develop an experimental treatment 20 years ago that now could save my life. I believed in the hard currency of his intelligence and his research.

Beyond that, I had no idea where to draw the line between spiritual belief and science. But I knew this much: I believed in belief, for its own shining sake. To believe in the face of utter hopelessness, every article of evidence to the contrary, to ignore apparent catastrophe— what other choice was there? We do it every day, I realized. We are so much stronger than we imagine, and belief is one of the most valiant and long-lived human characteristics. To believe, when all along we humans know that nothing can cure the briefness of this life, that there is no remedy for our basic mortality, that is a form of bravery.

To continue believing in yourself, believing in the doctors, believing in the treatment, believing in whatever I chose to believe in, that was the most important thing, I decided. It had to be.

Without belief, we would be left with nothing but an overwhelming doom, every single day. And it will beat you. I didn't fully see, until the cancer, how we fight every day against the creeping negatives of the world, how we struggle daily against the slow lapping of cynicism. Dispiritedness and disappointment, these were the real perils of life, not some sudden illness or cataclysmic millennium doomsday. I knew now why people fear cancer: because it is a slow and inevitable death, it *is* the very definition of cynicism and loss of spirit.

So, I believed.

WHEN YOU CAN'T REMEMBER SOMETHING, THERE'S A reason why. I've blocked out much of what I thought and felt the morning of my brain surgery, but one thing I remember clearly is the date, October 25th, because when it was over I was so glad to be alive.

My mother and Och and Bill Stapleton came into my room at 6 A.M. to wake me up, and various nurses came by to prepare me for the surgery. Before you undergo a brain operation, you have a memory test. The doctors say, "We're going to tell you three simple words, and try to remember them for as long as you can." Some brain-tumor patients have lapses and can't remember what they were told ten minutes ago. If the tumor has affected you, it's the little things that you can't recall.

A nurse said, "Ball, pin, driveway. At some point we will ask you to repeat these words."

It could be 30 minutes later, or it could be three hours, but I would be asked for them eventually, and if I forgot, that would mean big trouble. I didn't want anyone to think I had a problem—I was still trying to prove I wasn't really as sick as the medical experts thought. I was determined to remember those words, so they were all I thought about for several minutes: *Ball, pin, driveway. Ball, pin, driveway.*

A half hour later a doctor returned and asked me for the words.

"Ball, pin, driveway," I said, confidently.

It was time to go to surgery. I was wheeled down the hall, with my mother walking part of the way, until we turned into the surgical room, where a team of masked nurses and doctors was waiting for me. They propped me up on the operating table, as the anesthesiologist began the job of administering the knockout punch.

For some reason, I felt chatty.

"Did you guys ever see the movie *Malice?*" I asked.

A nurse shook her head.

Enthusiastically, I launched into a summary of the plot: Alec Baldwin plays this gifted but arrogant surgeon who is sued for malpractice, and at his trial, a lawyer accuses him of suffering from something called the God Complex—believing that he is infallible.

Baldwin gives a great speech in his own defense—but then he incriminates himself. He describes the tension and the pressure of surgery when a patient is lying on a table and he has to make split-second decisions that determine life or death.

"At that moment, gentlemen," he declares, "I don't *think* I'm God. I *am* God."

I finished the story, doing a dead-on imitation of Alec Baldwin.

My next word was "Unnnnnhhh."

And I passed straight out from the anesthesia.

The thing about that speech is that there is an element of truth in it, absolute truth. As I passed into unconsciousness, my doctors controlled my future. They controlled my ability to sleep, and to reawaken. For that period of time, they were the ultimate beings. My doctors were my Gods.

Anesthesia was like a blackout: one moment I was cognizant, and the next moment I didn't even exist. The anesthesiologist, in testing the levels, brought me to consciousness just briefly before the surgery began. As I woke up, I realized that the surgery was not over; in fact, it had not even gotten under way, and I was furious. I said, woozily, "Damn it, let's get started."

I heard Shapiro's voice say, "Everything's fine," and I blacked out again.

All I know about the surgery, of course, is what Dr. Shapiro related to me later. I was on the table for roughly six hours. He made the incision and went about the job of removing the lesions. As soon as he scraped them away, he gave them to a pathologist, who put them right under a microscope.

By examining the tissue immediately, they could tell what sort of cancer it was and how likely it was to spread. If it was a lively and aggressive form of cancer, then there was a likelihood that more of it would be found.

But the pathologist looked up from the microscope, surprised, and said, "It's necrotic tissue."

"They're dead?" Shapiro said.

"They're dead," the technician said.

It was impossible to say that every cell was dead, of course. But they had every appearance of being lifeless and nonthreatening. It was the best possible news, because it meant they weren't spreading. What killed them? I don't know, and neither do the doctors. Some necrotic tissue isn't uncommon.

Shapiro went straight from the surgery to find my mother, and said, "He's in the recovery room and doing well." He explained that the tissue was necrotic, which meant there probably wasn't any more of it, they had gotten it all.

"It went much better than we ever expected," Shapiro said.

I WOKE UP . . . SLOWLY . . . IT WAS VERY BRIGHT AND . . . and someone was speaking to me.

I'm alive.

I opened my eyes. I was in the recovery room, and Scott Shapiro was bending over me. Once a doctor has cracked your skull and performed brain surgery, and then put you back together again, there is a moment of truth. No matter how good the surgeon, he waits anxiously to see if everything moves, and whether the patient is properly responsive.

"Do you remember me?" he said.

"You're my doctor," I said.

"What's my name?"

"Scott Shapiro."

"Can you tell me your name?"

"Lance Armstrong," I said. "And I can kick your ass on a bike any day."

I began to fade back to sleep, but as my eyes closed, I saw the same doctor who had tested my memory.

"Ball, pin, driveway," I said.

I dropped back into the black dreamless bottomless anesthetic sleep.

When I awoke again, I was in a dim, quiet room, in intensive care. I just lay there for a moment, fighting the haze of anesthesia. It was terribly dim, and quiet. I wanted to leave. *Move.*

I moved in the sheets.

"He's awake," a nurse said.

I threw a leg over the bed.

"Stay down!" a nurse said. "What are you doing?"

"I'm getting up," I said.

I started to rise.

Move. If you can still move, you aren't sick.

"You can't get up yet," she said. "Lie down."

I lay back down.

"I'm hungry," I announced.

As I became more fully conscious, I realized that my head was completely wrapped in gauze and bandages. My senses seemed wrapped up, too, probably a result of the anesthesia and the IV tubes twining all over me. I had tubes in my nose, and a catheter running up my leg and into my penis. I was exhausted, drained to the absolute center of my being.

But I was starving. I was used to my three square meals a day, thanks to my mother. I thought of heaping hot plates of food, with gravy. I hadn't eaten anything in hours, and my last meal had been some kind of cereal. Cereal wasn't a meal. I mean, come on. That was a snack.

A nurse fed me a plate of scrambled eggs.

"Can I see my mother?" I said.

After a bit, my mother came in quietly and held my hand. I understood how she felt, how offended her sense of motherhood was by seeing me like that. I had come from the same skin as hers, the physical matter that made me, every particle down to the last proton in the fingernail on my smallest finger, belonged to her, and when I was a baby she had counted my breaths in the night. She thought she had gotten me through the hard part, before this.

"I love you," I said. "I love my life, and you gave it to me, and I owe you so much for that."

I wanted to see my friends, too. The nurses allowed them to come in, two or three at a time. I had been careful to seem confident before the surgery, but now that it was over, I didn't need to put up a front anymore, to hide how relieved I was and how vulnerable I felt. Och came in, and then Chris, and they took my hands, and it felt good to let go of some things, to show them how afraid I had been. "I'm not done," I said. "I'm still here."

I was dazed, but I was aware of everyone who came into the room, and could sense what they were feeling. Kevin's voice was choked with emotion. He was deeply upset, and I wanted to reassure him.

"Why do you sound so serious?" I teased him.

He just squeezed my hand.

"I know," I said. "You don't like seeing your big brother all beat-up."

As I lay there, listening to the murmurs of my friends, two conflicting emotions welled up in me. First, I felt a giant wave of gratitude. But then I felt a second wave, of anger, and that second swell of feeling met the first one like two waves colliding. I was alive, and I was mad, and I couldn't feel the one without feeling the other. I was alive enough to *be* mad. I was fighting mad, swinging mad, mad in general, mad at being in a bed, mad at having bandages around my head, mad at the tubes that tied me down. So mad I was beside myself. So mad I almost began to cry.

Chris Carmichael grabbed my hand. By now Chris and I had been together for six years, and there was nothing we couldn't tell each other, no feeling we couldn't admit to.

"How you doing?" he asked.

"I'm great."

"Okay. Now, really, how do you feel?"

"Chris, I'm doing great."

"Yeah, right."

"Chris, you don't understand," I said, starting to cry. "I'm glad about this. You know what? I *like* it like this. I like the odds stacked against me, they always have been, and I don't know any other way. It's such *bullshit,* but it's just one more thing I'm going to overcome. This is the only way I want it."

————

I REMAINED IN THE ICU OVERNIGHT. AT ONE POINT, A nurse handed me a tube and told me to breathe into it. The tube was attached to a gauge with a little red ball, and it was supposed to measure my lung capacity, to make sure the anesthesia hadn't done something to my lungs.

"Breathe into this," the nurse said. "Now, don't worry if you only get the ball up one or two notches."

"Lady, are you kidding me?" I said. "I do this for a living. Give me that fucker."

I grabbed the tube and breathed into it. The ball shot straight to the top. If it had had a bell, it would have gone PING!

I handed it back to her.

"Don't ever bring that thing in here again," I said. "My lungs are fine."

The nurse left without a word. I looked over at my mother. My mother has always known I have a mouth on me, and I figured I would hear from her because I had been so rude to the nurse. But my mother was grinning as if I had just won another triple crown. She saw it for herself: nothing was wrong with me. I was right back to normal.

"That's my boy," she said. "Son, you're going to be just fine."

THE NEXT MORNING I RETURNED TO MY REGULAR room to begin chemotherapy. I would stay in the hospital for six more days, receiving treatment, and the results would be critical.

I was still reading up on cancer, and I knew that if the chemo didn't arrest the disease, I might not make it, no matter how successful the brain surgery had been. All of the books spelled out my status succinctly. "Patients whose disease progresses during cisplatin-based chemotherapy have a poor prognosis with any form of treatment," one book said.

I flipped through an academic study on testicular cancer that listed various treatments and survival rates, and in the margins I made calculations and notes with a pencil. But still, it all came down to the same thing: "Failure to achieve complete remission with initial chemotherapy is associated with a poor survival," the article stated. So there it was in a nutshell: the chemo would either work—or not.

There was nothing to do but sit in bed and let the toxins seep into my body—and be abused by nurses with needles. One thing they don't tell you about hospitals is how they violate you. It's like your body is no longer your own, it belongs to the nurses and the doctors, and they are free to prod you and force things into your veins and various openings. The catheter was the worst; it ran up my leg into my groin, and having it put in and then taken out again was agonizing. In a way, the small, normal procedures were the most awful part of illness. At least for the brain surgery I'd been knocked out, but for everything else, I was fully awake, and there were bruises and scabs and needle marks all over me, in the backs of my hands, my arms, my groin. When I was awake, the nurses ate me alive.

Shapiro came by and said the surgery had been a complete success: they had removed the lesions, and there was no sign of more. I had no intellectual or cognitive disturbances, and my coordination was fine. "Now it's a matter of hoping like hell it doesn't come back," he said.

TWENTY-FOUR HOURS AFTER BRAIN SURGERY, I WENT out to dinner.

As Shapiro promised, I rebounded from the operation quickly. That evening, my mother, Lisa, Och, Chris, and Bill helped me out of bed to take me across the street to the Rock Bottom Restaurant and Brewery. Shapiro hadn't told us there was anything we could or couldn't do, and I wanted to stick to the nutritional plan, so I put on a stocking cap to hide my bandages and we left the hospital. Bill had even gotten us tickets to an Indiana Pacers NBA game, and offered to take me, but that was a bit much. I did okay through most of the dinner, but toward the dessert I didn't feel so good, so we skipped the game and I went back to my sickbed.

The next day, Shapiro came by the room to remove the bandages from my wounds. As he unwound the gauze, I could feel the fabric tearing away from the staples, as though something was nipping at me. Then he pulled it off. I looked in the mirror. I had staples running in curves across my scalp, like two circled zippers. Shapiro said, "I've done my part."

I studied the staples in the mirror. I knew that Shapiro had used titanium screws to put my skull back together beneath my skin. Titanium is an alloy used in some lighter-weight bikes. "Maybe it'll make me climb better," I joked.

Shapiro became a good friend, and he continued to drop by my room to see how I was doing over the next months of treatments. It was always good to see him, no matter how sleepy or nauseated I was.

Larry Einhorn returned from Australia, and visited me, too. He was terribly busy, but he made time to see me periodically, and participated in my treatment. He, like Dr. Nichols and Dr. Shapiro, was one of those physicians who make you understand the meaning of the word "healer." I began to think that they knew more about life and death than most people; they had a view of humanity that others didn't, because they surveyed so much emotional landscape. They not only saw people live and die, they witnessed how we handled those two circumstances, unmasked, with all of our irrational optimism and fear and incredible strength, on a daily basis.

"I've seen wonderful, positive people not make it in the end," Dr. Einhorn said. "And some of the most miserable, ornery people survive to resume their ornery lives."

I BEGAN TO GET GOOD NEWS. NONE OF MY SPONSORS was bailing out on me. Bill and I braced for the calls to start coming in, but they never did. As the days went on, all we heard from Nike, Giro, Oakley, and Milton-Bradley were words of support.

My relationship with Nike went back to when I was a high-school runner and a triathlete, and thought their progressive messages were cool and their athletes the most hip. But I never figured I'd be a Nike guy, because I didn't play in Dodger Stadium, or Soldiers Field, or Roland Garros—instead I played on the roads of France, Belgium, and Spain. Still, when my career took off, I asked Bill Stapleton to see if he could get me a Nike deal because I yearned to belong to their company. In 1996, right before I was diagnosed, Nike offered me an endorsement contract to wear their shoes and gloves.

I instantly became close friends with Scott MacEachern, the Nike representative assigned to cycling, and so it was no accident that he was one of the first people I told about my cancer. In my conversation with Scott that night after returning home from Dr. Reeves' office, all the horrible emotions I had suppressed broke loose. I started crying as I told Scott the whole story, about the pain in my groin, and the shock of the chest X ray. After a while, I stopped crying. There was a moment of silence on the other end of the line, and then Scott spoke calmly, almost casually.

"Well, don't worry about us," he said. "We're with you."

It was a tiny hopeful seed of a feeling; maybe I wasn't totally ruined and alone. Scott was true to his word; Nike didn't desert me. As I got sicker, it meant everything. What's more, my other sponsors responded the same way. One by one, I heard the same sentiments from Giro, Oakley, and Milton-Bradley.

They would not only stay with me, something even more remarkable happened. Bill was desperate over the matter of my health coverage. He had looked for some way I could claim coverage, but it seemed hopeless.

Bill picked up the phone and called Mike Parnell, the CEO of Oakley. He explained what had happened. Hesitantly, Bill asked Mike if they could help me.

Mike said he would arrange for me to be covered.

Suddenly, I had reason for optimism. But then the health care provider balked; I had a preexisting condition and therefore they were not obliged to cover my cancer treatments.

Mike Parnell picked up the phone and called the provider. He informed them that if they did not cover my medical treatments, his entire firm would take its business elsewhere.

"Cover him," he said.

The provider still balked.

"I don't think you understand what I just said," Mike said.

They covered me.

I'll spend the rest of my life trying to adequately convey what it meant to me, and I'll be an Oakley, Nike, and Giro athlete for as long as I live. They paid my contracts in full, every single one—even though each of them had the right to terminate the deal—and none of them ever so much as asked me about when I would ride a bike again. In fact, when I went to them and said, "Hey, I've started this cancer foundation [more about that later] and I need some money to stage a charity bike race," every single one of them stepped forward to help. So don't talk to me about the cold world of business. Cancer was teaching me daily to examine my fellow human beings more deeply, to throw out my previous assumptions and oversimplifications.

The good news continued through that week in the hospital. After a couple of days of chemo, my blood counts improved. The markers were falling, which meant that the cancer was reacting to the drugs. I still had a long hard pull ahead of me, and I was beginning to feel the side effects Nichols had warned me of. As I approached the end of the week, the euphoria of coming through brain surgery wore off, and the sickness of ifosfamide took over. It gave me a constant poisoned sensation and left me so weak that all I wanted to do was stare at the wall or sleep. And this was just the start of it; there were two more cycles yet to come.

Seven days after the brain surgery, I went home. I would be back in the hospital soon enough. But at least I was beginning to talk this thing down to size.

six

CHEMO

THE QUESTION WAS, WHICH WOULD THE CHEMO kill first: the cancer, or me? My life became one long IV drip, a sickening routine: if I wasn't in pain I was vomiting, and if I wasn't vomiting, I was thinking about what I had, and if I wasn't thinking about what I had, I was wondering when it was going to be over. That's chemo for you.

The sickness was in the details, in the nasty asides of the treatment. Cancer was a vague sense of unwellness, but chemo was an endless series of specific horrors, until I began to think the cure was as bad as, or worse than, the disease. What a casual bystander associates with cancer—loss of hair, a sickly pallor, a wasting away—are actually the side effects of the treatment. Chemo was a burning in my veins, a matter of being slowly eaten from the inside out by a destroying river of pollutants until I didn't have an eyelash left to bat. Chemo was a continuous cough, hacking up black chunks of mysterious, tar-like matter from deep in my chest. Chemo was a constant, doubling-over need to go to the bathroom.

To cope with it, I imagined I was coughing out the burned-up tumors. I envisioned the chemo working on them, singeing them, and expelling them from my system. When I went to the bathroom I endured the acid sting in my groin by telling myself I was peeing out dead cancer cells. I suppose that's how you do it. They've got to go somewhere, don't they? I was coughing up cancer, pissing it out, getting rid of it every way I knew how.

I had no life other than chemo. My old forms of keeping dates and time fell by the wayside, substituted for by treatment regimens. I spent every major holiday that fall and winter either on a chemo cycle or recovering from one. I spent Halloween night with an IV in me and passed out bags of candy to the nurses. I went home for Thanksgiving and recuperated on my couch while my mother tried to persuade me to eat a few bites of turkey. I slept 10 to 12 hours a night, and when I was awake, I was in a funk that felt like a combination of jet lag and a hangover.

Chemo has a cumulative effect; I underwent four cycles in the space of three months, and toxins built up in my body with each phase. At first it wasn't so bad; by the end of the second set of treatments I just felt sickish and constantly sleepy. I would check into the Indianapolis medical center on a Monday, and take five hours of chemo for five straight days, finishing on Friday. When I wasn't on chemo, I was attached to a 24-hour IV drip of saline and a chemical protectant to shield my immune system from the most toxic effects of ifosfamide, which is particularly damaging to the kidneys and the bone marrow.

But by the third cycle I was on my hands and knees fighting nausea. A wave would come over me, and I'd feel as if all of my vital organs had gone bad inside my body. By the fourth cycle—the highest number prescribed for cancer patients, and only in the most severe cases—I was in the fetal position, retching around the clock.

Dr. Nichols offered to let me do the chemo as an outpatient in Austin. "You can do it at home and we'll consult," he said. But I insisted on commuting to Indianapolis so that I could be constantly monitored.

"If I get sicker, I want you to be able to see it," I told him. "And if I get better, I want you to see that, too."

Chemo didn't look like anything. It was hard to believe that a substance so deadly could appear so innocuous. The drugs came in three clear plastic 50cc bags, labeled with my name, the date, the dose, and the volume of fluid. The silvery clear liquids floated harmlessly in their plastic containers, without any precipitate. They could just as easily have been bags of sugar water. The giveaway was the pair of heavy latex gloves the nurse used to handle the bags, and the stamp that said "Hazardous Materials." The nurse would insert tubing into a bag, and infuse it through another tube into my catheter, and thus into my bloodstream. One bag took an hour, another took 90 minutes, and the last one took 30.

But those liquids were so destructive they could literally evaporate all of the blood in my body. I felt like my veins were being scoured out. The medical explanation for the sensation I experienced was myelosuppression, the most frequent and severe side effect of chemotherapy, which is the inhibition of red blood cell production and maturation. Chemo weakens your blood. During the third cycle, my hematocrit—the percentage of total blood volume flowing through my body—fell to less than 25, and the normal count is 46. Ironically, I was given a red blood cell booster called Epogen (EPO). In any other situation, taking EPO would get me in trouble with the International Cycling

Union and the International Olympic Committee, because it's considered performance-enhancing. But in my case, the EPO was hardly that. It was the only thing that kept me alive.

Chemo doesn't just kill cancer—it kills healthy cells, too. It attacked my bone marrow, my muscle, my teeth, and the linings of my throat and my stomach, and left me open to all kinds of infections. My gums bled. I got sores in my mouth. And of course I lost my appetite, which was a potentially serious problem. Without enough protein, I wouldn't be able to rebuild tissue after chemo had eaten through my skin, my hair, and my fingernails.

Mornings were hardest. I would finish a treatment shortly before dinner. I'd try to eat something, and then I'd lie in bed, watching television or visiting with my friends. The drugs would penetrate into my system through the night, and I would wake up the next day in a thick cloud of nausea. There was only one thing I could tolerate: apple fritters from the hospital cafeteria. It was strange, but the crispy dough, the icy sugar, and the jam-like apple filling were soothing on my tongue and stomach.

Every morning Jim Ochowicz would show up with a box full of them. He'd sit at the foot of the bed, and we'd eat them together. Och brought me those fritters every single day, long past the point when I was capable of actually eating them.

Chemo was lonely. My mother finally went home to Plano after the brain surgery; she had exhausted her vacation time and couldn't afford to take an unpaid leave. She hated to go; she thought that just by being there she could make a difference.

When I was in high school she used to believe that if she kept watch over me, nothing bad could happen to me. When a norther would hit Plano and the streets iced over, my buddies and I used to go to the Plano East parking lot, tie a snow disc to the back of a car, and tow each other around. My mother would drive up and watch us from her car. "I feel like if I'm here I can keep you from getting hurt," she said. She felt the same way about chemo, but she didn't have a choice.

Och took her place, my surrogate parent and my most constant bedside companion. He made the long drive over from Wisconsin and sat with me for every cycle, day in and day out. Och understood the slow, corrosive effects of the chemo on a patient's spirit, because he had lost his father to cancer. He knew how demoralizing the treatment was, and how tedious, and he tirelessly sought ways to divert me. He taught me how to play Hearts, and he sat next to my bed, dealing the cards for hours on end, with Bill and Lisa making up a foursome. He read the newspaper and the mail to me when I was too sick to read it myself.

He took me for walks around the hospital, wheeling my IV pole, while we talked about everything from cycling to Internet stocks. One afternoon, we talked about death. We sat in the sun on a bench outside the medical center. "Och, I don't feel ready to go, I think I'm supposed to live," I said. "I'm not afraid to die if I have to. But I'm still not convinced I can't beat this thing."

But chemo felt like a kind of living death. I would lie in bed half-asleep, and lose track of time, including whether it was day or night—and I didn't like that. It was disorienting and made me feel as if things were slipping out of joint, getting away from me. Och created a routine so I could gauge the time. He brought my apple fritters for breakfast, and chatted with me until I dozed off in the middle of a sentence. My chin would fall on my chest, and Och would tiptoe out of the room. A few hours later he would come back with a plate of vegetables for lunch, or a sandwich he had bought outside the hospital. After lunch, we would play cards until I passed out again, my head nodding and my eyelids fluttering. Och would take the cards out of my hand and put them back in the deck, and tiptoe softly out.

Bill and Lisa were also there for every cycle, and others floated in and out of town; loyal sponsors and old friends took turns showing up. Och, Bill, and Lisa were the core group, my social chairmen. Every evening, the three of them would bring me some dinner, or, if I felt well enough, I would walk with them down to the cafeteria, dragging my little IV cart behind me. But I was never really up for the meal; it was just to break the monotony. Afterward we'd watch some TV until I began to doze, and then they would leave me at about 7 P.M., and I would be alone for the night.

It became a ritual for the three of them to eat together, along with any other visitors who had come to see me, like Chris Carmichael or Scott MacEachern. They would go to the Palomino Euro Bistro, or to a great old steakhouse named St. Elmo, and afterward they'd go to the bar at the Canterbury Hotel and smoke cigars. It was everything I would have enjoyed, if I hadn't been sick. In the evening when they got ready to leave, I'd say accusingly, "You guys are going to drink your asses off again, aren't you?"

WHEN LATRICE CAME IN TO GIVE ME THE CHEMO, NO matter how sick I was, I would sit up and be as attentive as I could.

"What are you putting in me?" I'd ask. "What's the mix?"

By now I could read a chest X ray as well as any doctor could, and I knew all the terms and anti-nausea dosages. I quizzed LaTrice on them, and told her what felt better or worse from the standpoint of nausea. I'd say, "Try a little less of this." Or, "Give me a little more of that."

I was not a compliant cancer patient. I was salty, aggressive, and pestering. I personalized the disease. "The Bastard," I called it. I made it my enemy, my challenge. When LaTrice said, "Drink five glasses of

water in a day," I drank fifteen, draining them one after the other until
the water ran down my chin.

Chemo threatened to deprive me of my independence and self-
determination, and that was galling. I was tied to an IV pole for 24
hours a day, and it was a hard thing for me to cede control to my nurses
and doctors. I insisted on behaving as if I was a full participant in the
cure. I followed the blood work and the X rays closely, and badgered
LaTrice as if I were the Grand Inquisitor.

"Who are my nurses today, LaTrice?"

"What's that drug called, LaTrice?"

"What does that one do, LaTrice?"

I questioned her constantly, as if somehow I was the one in charge.
LaTrice coordinated the chemo with the nurses on the unit: she made
out my schedule and the anti-emetic regime, and managed the symptoms. I kept track of everything, I knew exactly what I was supposed
to get, and when, and I noticed every slight variation in the routine.

LaTrice adopted an air of exaggerated patience with me. This was
a typical day for her:

"What dose am I getting, LaTrice?" I'd ask.

"What's that based on?"

"Am I getting the same thing as yesterday?"

"Why am I getting a different one?"

"What time do we start, LaTrice?"

"When do I finish, LaTrice?"

I made a game out of timing the completion of treatments. I would
look at my wristwatch, and stare at the IV bags as they emptied into
my body by droplets. I tried to calculate the rate of drip, and time the
end of the treatment down to the last second.

"When, exactly, is my last drop, LaTrice?"

As the time went on, LaTrice and I developed a kidding relationship. I accused her of withholding anti-emetics out of cruelty. They were all that kept me from cringing with illness from the chemo. But I could only have a dose every four hours, so I'd hassle LaTrice for more.

"I can't give you more," she'd say. "You got it three hours ago, you've just got an hour left."

"Come on, LaTrice. You run the show around here. You know you can do it. You just don't want to."

Every once in a while, I'd give in to the retching, and vomit so hard I thought I might pass out. "I feel much better now," I'd tell LaTrice, sarcastically, once I was through.

Sometimes food triggered me, especially breakfast food. Finally, I stopped them from bringing the tray at all. One morning I stared balefully at a plateful of eggs that seemed hopelessly gooey and toast that looked like plasterboard, and I exploded.

"What is this shit?" I said. "LaTrice, would *you* eat this? Look at this. You *feed* this to people? Can someone please get me something to *eat?*"

"Lance, you can have whatever you want," LaTrice said serenely.

LaTrice gave as good as she got. She would tease me back, even when I was too ill to laugh.

"Is it me, Lance?" LaTrice would ask with exaggerated sympathy. "Am I what's making you sick?"

I would just grin, soundlessly, and retch again. We were becoming friends, comrades in chemo. Between cycles I went home to Austin for two-week rest periods to regain my strength, and LaTrice always called to check up on me and make sure I was drinking my fluids. The chemo could damage my urinary tract, so she was always after me to hydrate. One night she called when I was fooling around in my carport with a present from Oakley. It was a small remote-control car made out of titanium that could do up to 70 miles per hour.

"What's that loud buzzing noise?" she said.

"I'm in my garage," I said.

"What are you doing?" she said.

"I'm playing with my toy car," I said.

"Of course you are," she said.

ONE DAY I NOTICED STRANGE MARKS ON MY SKIN, AL-most like faint brown stains. They were chemo burns.

The drugs were scorching my tissues from the inside out, leaving patches of discoloration on my flesh. By now I was well into the third cycle, and I didn't look like the same person. My physique was shot, compared to the one I entered the hospital with. I took hobbling walks around the floor to get a little exercise, pushing my IV pole, and I remember looking down at myself in my gown. It was as though my body was being steadily diminished: my muscles were smaller, and flaccid. *This is the real McCoy,* I thought. *This is what it means to be sick.*

"I need to stay in shape," I'd murmur. "I need to stay in shape."

I kept losing weight, no matter how hard I tried not to. I didn't have much to lose to begin with—I had a very low percent of body fat, and the toxins ate away at me like a school of fish, nibbling. "LaTrice, I'm losing weight," I'd lament. "What can I do? Look at my muscles! Look what's happening to me. I need to ride. I've got to get toned back up."

"Lance, it's *chemo,*" LaTrice would say, in that supremely tolerant way. "You're going to lose, it's automatic. Chemo patients lose weight."

I couldn't bear to stay in bed, dormant. As I lay in the sheets, doing nothing, I felt like something that had washed up on a beach.

"Can I exercise, LaTrice?"

"Do you have a gym here, LaTrice?"

"Lance, this is a *hospital,*" she'd say, with that great sighing forbearance of hers. "However, for patients who have to stay with us for a long time, and for people like you, we do have stationary bikes."

"Can I do that?" I shot back.

LaTrice asked Nichols for an okay to let me use the gym, but Nichols was reluctant. My immune system was almost nonexistent, and I wasn't in any condition to work out.

For all of her mocking exasperation with me, LaTrice seemed to sympathize with my restless urge to move. One afternoon I was scheduled for an MRI scan to check my brain, but the machines were fully booked, so LaTrice sent me over to the nearby children's hospital, Riley. An underground tunnel of about a mile attached the two facilities, and the usual way to transport patients between them was either in an ambulance, or in a wheelchair via the tunnel.

But I was determined to walk to Riley, not ride. I informed the nurse who showed up with a wheelchair, "No way I'm getting in that thing." I told her we would be taking the tunnel to Riley on foot, even if it meant walking all night. LaTrice didn't say a word. She just shook her head as I set off. The nurse dragged my IV cart behind me.

I shuffled slowly through the tunnel, there and back. I looked like a stooped, limping old man. The round-trip took over an hour. By the time I got back to my bed, I was exhausted and damp with sweat, but I was triumphant.

"You just had to do it different," LaTrice said, and smiled.

It became the biggest fight of all just to move. By the fifth straight day of my third cycle of chemo, I was no longer able to take my walks around the ward. I had to lie in bed for a full day until I regained enough strength to go home. An attendant turned up Sunday morning with a wheelchair and offered me a ride to the lobby to check out. But I refused to give in to it. I turned it down, angrily.

"No way," I said. "I'm walking out of here."

THE FRENCHMAN HOVERED OVER MY HOSPITAL BED, attempting to present me with a $500 bottle of red wine as a token of his esteem. I stared at him from the depths of my narcotic haze, half-conscious and too nauseated to respond. I did have the presence of mind to wonder why anyone would waste an expensive Bordeaux on a cancer patient.

Alain Bondue was the director of the Cofidis racing organization, and he had come to pay what appeared to be a social call. But I was in no shape to make polite conversation; I was in the late throes of my third cycle of chemo, and I was deathly pale with dark circles under my eyes. I had no hair or eyebrows. Bondue spent a couple of awkward minutes pledging the support of the team, and then took his leave.

"Lance, we love you," he said. "We're going to take care of you, I promise."

With that, he said goodbye, and I squeezed his hand. But as he left my bedside, Bondue gestured to Bill Stapleton—he wanted him to come outside for a conversation. Bill followed Bondue into the hallway, and abruptly, Bondue told Bill he had come to discuss some business matters, and they needed to go someplace private for a meeting.

Stapleton and Bondue and a third man, a friend named Paul Sherwen who spoke French and offered to help interpret, gathered in a small, dimly lit conference room in the hotel across the street from the hospital. Bondue began to chain-smoke as he explained to Bill in French that, regrettably, Cofidis would be forced to renegotiate my contract because of my illness. My agreement with the team was for $2.5 million over two years—but that would no longer be possible.

Bill shook his head in confusion. "I'm sorry?" he said. Cofidis had publicly pledged to stand by me while I fought the illness, he said. Surely this wasn't the time to discuss contracts, not in the middle of my chemotherapy.

"We love Lance; we want to take care of Lance," Bondue said in French. "But you have to understand this is a cultural thing, and people in France don't understand how somebody can get paid when they're not working."

Bill was stunned. He said, "I don't believe what I'm hearing."

Bondue pointed out that my contract had a clause stating I was required to pass a medical examination. Obviously, I was in no condition to do that. Therefore Cofidis had the right to cancel the contract. They were offering to renegotiate, which they felt was generous under the circumstances. They wanted to honor part of it, but not all. If I didn't accept the new terms they offered, they would force me to undergo the medical exam, and terminate the contract in its entirety.

Bill stood up, looked across the table, and said, "Fuck you."

Bondue was startled.

Bill said it again. "Fuck you. I cannot believe you came all the way here at a time like this, and you want me to go back in there and tell him that now."

Bill was beside himself—not so much that Cofidis would try to extricate themselves from the contract, which they had the right to do, but at the timing, and the backhandedness of it. Cofidis had made a statement to the world that they would stick with me, and they had reaped the favorable press for it, but behind closed doors was another matter. Bill was fiercely protective of me, and he flatly refused to raise the subject with me while I was in the midst of chemo.

"I'm not doing it," Bill said. "I'm not interested in talking about this, not right now. Do whatever you guys want to do, and let it play out in the court of public opinion."

Bondue was unmoved. Legally, he intoned, surely Bill knew that we didn't have a leg to stand on. Cofidis had the right to terminate that very day. Instantly.

"You understand it's subject to the medical exam," Bondue said again.

Bill said, "Are you going to send a doctor over here? Are you going to send a doctor over here to do an exam?"

"Well, we might have to," Bondue said.

"Great," Bill said. "I'll have all the television cameras there, and you guys knock yourselves out."

Bondue continued to insist that Cofidis was willing to keep me under some kind of contract—but only if a set of conditions was imposed. Bill calmed down and tried to persuade Bondue that, despite my appearance, I was getting better. Surely they could work something out? But Bondue was firm, and after two more hours, they had gotten nowhere. Finally, Bill stood up to leave. If Cofidis was pulling the rug out from under me while I was in the hospital, fine, he said, "I'll let the whole world know you abandoned him." Abruptly, Bill ended the meeting.

"Do whatever you have to do," he said.

Shaken, Bill came back to my hospital room. He had been gone for over three hours by now, so I knew something was wrong. As soon as the door to my room opened, I said, "What?"

"Nothing," Bill said. "Don't worry about it."

But I could see by the look on his face that he was upset, and I suspected I knew the reason why.

"What?"

"I don't know what to say," Bill said. "They want to renegotiate this thing, and they'll make you take a medical exam if they have to."

"Well, what are we going to do?"

"I've already told them to fuck off."

I thought about it. "Maybe we should just let it go," I said, tiredly.

I couldn't help wondering if the real reason for Bondue's trip was to appraise my health. I thought then, and I still think, that he came to the hospital with a choice to make: if I looked healthy, then he would take a positive attitude and let the deal stand, and if I looked very ill, he would take the hard-line approach and renegotiate or terminate. We felt that it was nothing more than a spy mission: see if Armstrong is dying. Apparently Bondue had taken one look at me and decided I was on my deathbed.

Bill was crushed, and apologetic. "I'm sorry to give you one more piece of bad news."

But I had more important things to dwell on than Cofidis. Don't get me wrong, I was worried about the money, and I was hurt by their timing, and by their halfhearted words of support. But on the other hand, I had a more immediate problem to concentrate on—not puking.

Bill said, "We'll stall. We'll keep negotiating." He thought if he could put them off until February, I might just be healthy enough to pass the medical exam. "We'll just see how this plays out," he said. I just grunted, too nauseated to really care. I didn't want to talk about it anymore.

Over the next three or four weeks, Cofidis pressed the issue and made it clear they weren't bluffing, they would have no problem subjecting me to a medical test. They would fly their own doctor over from France and cancel the entire contract. I continued to resist talking to Bill about it, because I was at my sickest point in the chemo cycles. But Bill sat down in my room one day and said, "Lance, they're serious." We had no choice but to accept whatever terms they gave me, he said.

In the end, Cofidis paid less than a third of the original two-year contract and required an out clause for themselves for 1998.

It felt like a vote of no confidence. It felt like they thought I was dying. I got the message Cofidis was sending: I was a dead man.

THE IRONY WAS, THE WORSE I FELT, THE BETTER I GOT.
That was the chemo for you.

By now I was so sick there were times I couldn't talk. So sick I
couldn't eat, couldn't watch TV, couldn't read my mail, couldn't even
speak to my mother on the phone. One afternoon she called me from
work. I whispered, "Mom, I'm going to have to talk to you another
time."

On the really bad days, I would lie on my side in bed, wrapped in
blankets, fighting the noxious roiling in my stomach and the fever
raging under my skin. I'd peek out from under the blankets and just
grunt.

The chemo left me so foggy that my memory of that time is
sketchy, but what I do know for sure is that at my sickest, I started to
beat the thing. The doctors would come in every morning with the
results of my latest blood-draw, and I began to get improved results.
One thing unique to the disease is that the marker levels are extremely
telling. We tracked every little fluctuation in my blood count; a slight
rise or downturn in an HCG or AFP marker was cause for either
concern or celebration.

The numbers had incredible import for my doctors and me. For instance, from October 2, when I was diagnosed, to October 14, when
the brain lesions were discovered, my HCG count had risen from
49,600 to 92,380. In the early days of my treatment, the doctors were
sober when they came into my room—I could tell they were suspending judgment.

But gradually they became more cheerful: the tumor markers began
to drop. Then they began to dive. Soon they were in a beautiful free
fall. In fact, the numbers were dropping so fast that the doctors were
a little taken aback. On a manila file folder, I kept a chart of my blood

markers. In just one three-week period in November, they fell from 92,000 to around 9,000.

"You're a responder," Nichols told me.

I had opened up a gap on the field. I knew that if I was going to be cured, that was the way it would go, with a big surging attack, just like in a race. Nichols said, "You're ahead of schedule." Those numbers became the highlight of each day; they were my motivator, my yellow jersey. The yellow jersey is the garment worn by the leader of the Tour de France to distinguish him from the rest of the field.

I began to think of my recovery like a time trial in the Tour. I was getting feedback from my team right behind me, and at every checkpoint the team director would come over the radio and say, "You're thirty seconds up." It made me want to go even faster. I began to set goals with my blood, and I would get psyched up when I met them. Nichols would tell me what they hoped to see in the next blood test, say a 50 percent drop. I would concentrate on that number, as if I could make the counts by mentally willing it. "They've split in half," Nichols would say, and I would feel like I had won something. Then one day he said, "They're a fourth of what they were."

I began to feel like I was winning the battle against the disease, and it made my cycling instincts kick in again. I wanted to tear the legs off cancer, the way I tore the legs off other riders on a hill. I was in a breakaway. "Cancer picked the wrong guy," I bragged to Kevin Livingston. "When it looked around for a body to hang out in, it made a big mistake when it chose mine. *Big* mistake."

One afternoon Dr. Nichols came into my room and read me a new number: my HCG was just 96. It was a slam-dunk. From now on it was just a matter of getting through the last and most toxic part of the treatments. I was almost well.

But I sure didn't feel like it. That was chemo for you.

BACK HOME IN TEXAS BETWEEN CHEMO CYCLES I WOULD gradually recover some strength, until I could begin to move again. I craved air and exercise.

Friends didn't let on how weak I had become. My out-of-town visitors must have been shocked at my pale, wasted, bald appearance, but they hid it well. Frankie Andreu came to stay with me for a week, and Chris Carmichael, and Eric Heiden, the great Olympic speedskater-turned-physician, and Eddy Merckx. They cooked for me, and took me on short walks and bicycle rides.

We'd leave my front door and go up a curving asphalt road that led to Mount Bonnell, a craggy peak above the Austin riverbank. Normally my friends had to sprint to keep up with my gear-mashing and hammering pedal strokes, but now we moved at a crawl. I would get winded on a completely flat road.

I don't think I had fully admitted the effect chemotherapy had on my body. I came into the cancer fight very brash and fit and confident, and I could see with each cycle that I was being drained somewhat, but I had no idea how incapacitating it truly was until I almost collapsed in a stranger's front yard.

Bike riding wasn't part of Dr. Nichols' recommendation. He didn't outright forbid it, but he said, "This is not the time to try to maintain or improve your fitness. Don't stress your body." I didn't listen—I was panicked at the idea that I would be so deconditioned by the chemo that I might never recover. My body was atrophying.

When I felt up to it, I would say to Kevin or Bart, "Let's go out and ride the bike." At first we would ride for anywhere from 30 to 50 miles, and I pictured myself as defiant, indefatigable, head down into the wind, racing along a road. But in reality the rides weren't like that at all; they were fairly desperate and feeble acts.

By the end of my treatments we would ride for half an hour, a simple loop around the neighborhood, and I told myself that as long as I could do that, I was staying in tolerable shape. But then two incidents showed me exactly how weakened I was. One afternoon I went out with Kevin, Bart, and Bart's fiancée, Barbara, and about halfway through the ride we reached a short, steep hill. I thought I was keeping up, but the truth was, my friends were being kind. In fact, they were moving so slowly they almost fell over sideways on their bikes. Sometimes they would pull ahead accidentally, and I would churn behind them, lamenting, "You're killing me." They were careful not to overwork me, so I had little concept of how fast or how slow we were going. I actually thought I was staying with them as we worked up the hill.

All of a sudden, a figure moved up on my left. It was a woman in her 50s on a heavy mountain bike, and she went right by me.

She cruised, without even breathing hard, while I puffed and chugged on my high-performance bike. I couldn't keep up with her. In cycling terms it's called getting dropped. I was giving it everything, and I couldn't stay with her.

You fool yourself. You fool yourself into thinking you might be riding faster and feeling better than you really are. Then a middle-aged woman on a mountain bike passes you, and you know exactly where you stand. I had to admit I was in bad shape.

It became an increasing struggle to ride my bike between the chemotherapy sessions, and I had to accept that it was no longer about fitness. Now I rode purely for the sake of riding—and that was new for me. To ride for only half an hour. I had never gone out for such a trivial amount of time on a bike.

I didn't love the bike before I got sick. It was simple for me: it was my job and I was successful at it. It was a means to an end, a way to

My mother looked even younger
than seventeen when she had me.
In a way, we grew up together.
(Courtesy of Linda Armstrong)

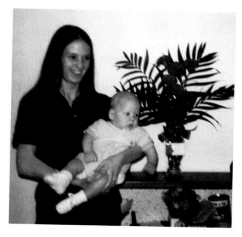

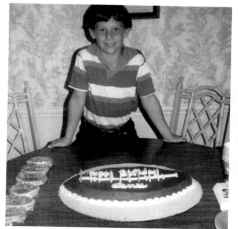

My ninth birthday, September 18,
1980. You can tell by my pressed shirt
and the size of the cake that my mom
made sure I didn't go without.
(Courtesy of Linda Armstrong)

At twelve, I was a swimming
prodigy, and a well-fed one. In
the kitchen with my best
friend and biggest supporter.
(Courtesy of Linda Armstrong)

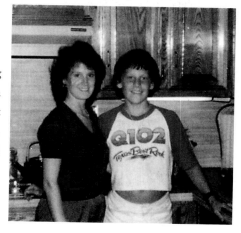

I was the youngest triathlete in the field. The older guys, like fellow triathlete Mark Allen, called me "Junior." *(Courtesy of Linda Armstrong)*

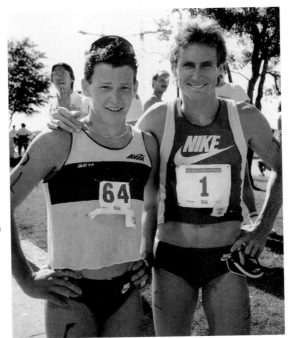

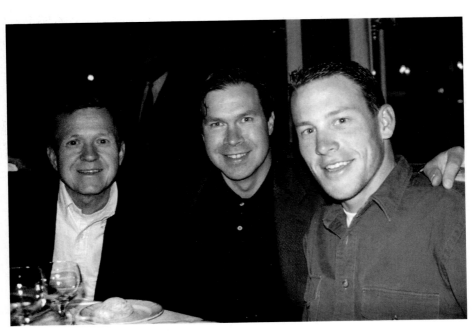

Before cancer, back in September 1995, I dined out with my friends J. T. Neal, from whom I rented my first apartment in Austin, complete with Longhorn over the mantel, and Jim Ochowicz, who taught me how to win on a bike. *(Courtesy of Linda Armstrong)*

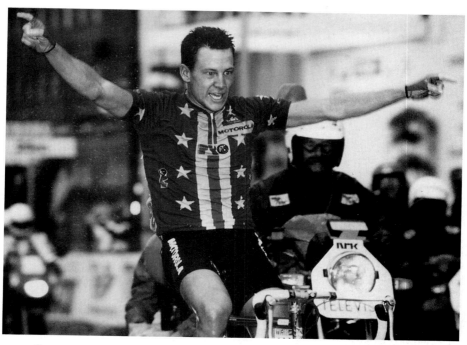

I was a twenty-one-year-old world champion in Oslo, 1993, and an angry young rider. I screamed as I launched my attack, and showboated across the finish line. *(Graham Watson)*

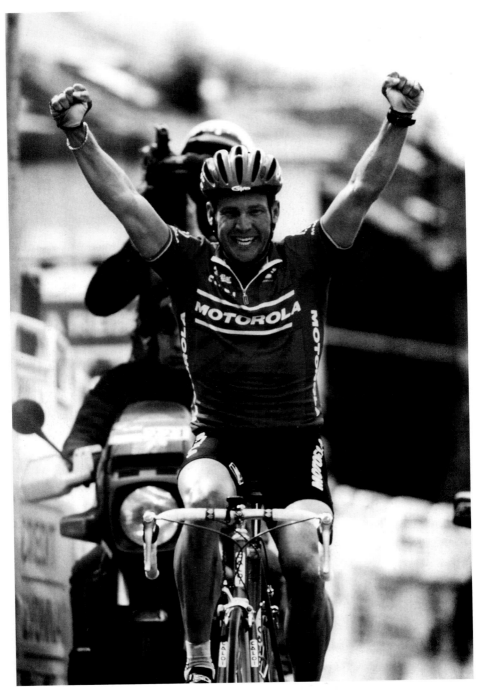

Y̲ou can see the obvious difference in my build pre-cancer in 1996, when I was the winner of the Fléche-Wallonne and a much heavier rider. *(Graham Watson)*

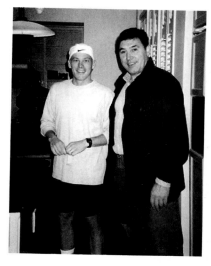

I was thin and sick between chemo treatments—but delighted to see my friend Eddy Merckx, the great Belgian five-time champion of the Tour de France, who came to Austin to cheer me up. Och is on the phone in the background. *(Courtesy of Linda Armstrong)*

Preparing for brain surgery: the dots on my head are to guide the surgeon to where the cancerous lesions are, while a nurse draws blood from the catheter in my chest. *(Courtesy of Linda Armstrong)*

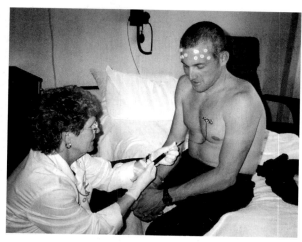

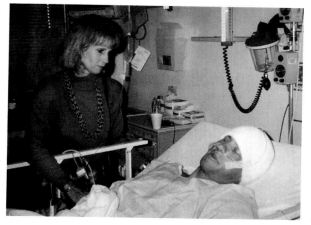

My mother was the first person I asked for after brain surgery. I remember being hungry and trying to get out of bed. *(Courtesy of Linda Armstrong)*

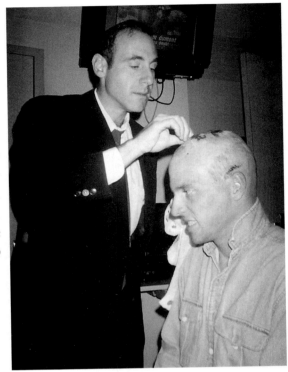

My neurosurgeon, Dr. Scott Shapiro, removing the bandages after surgery. My hair grew back in time, but I can still feel the scars. *(Courtesy of Linda Armstrong)*

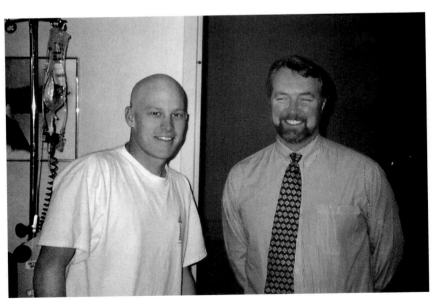

It must have been early in my chemo cycle, because I was able to laugh with my oncologist and friend, Dr. Craig Nichols. The bag and the IV pole followed me everywhere. *(Courtesy of Linda Armstrong)*

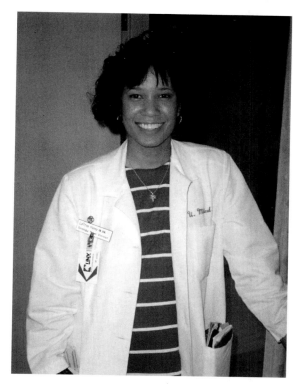

This is what a real angel looks like. LaTrice Haney, oncology nurse, Indiana University Medical Center.
(Susan Fox)

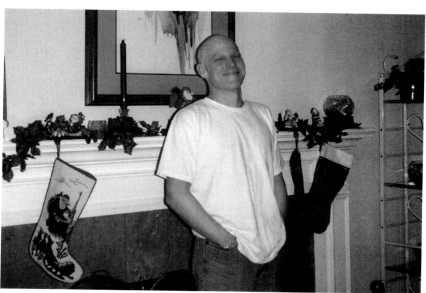

Christmas 1996, and I'm smiling because I'm still here.
(Courtesy of Linda Armstrong)

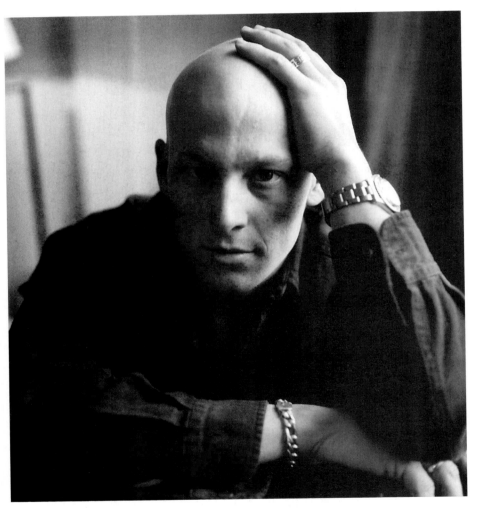

Remission: bald, scarred, and brooding. *(James Startt)*

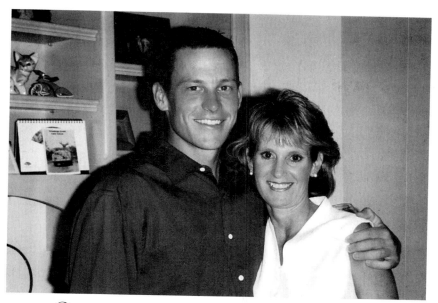

October 2, 1997, celebrating the one-year anniversary of my cancer diagnosis with my mother. *(Courtesy of Linda Armstrong)*

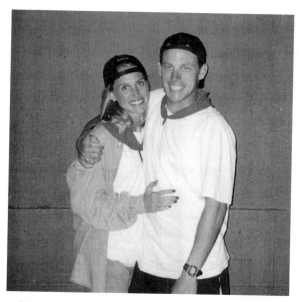

Me and Kik, pulling an all-nighter in Pamplona.
(Courtesy of Kristin Armstrong)

The view of Spain was different as a tourist . . . *(Courtesy of Kristin Armstrong)*

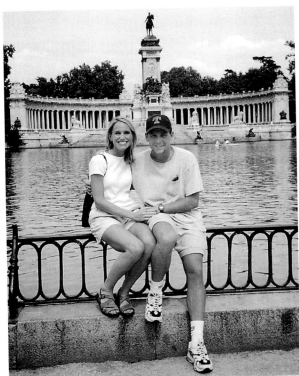

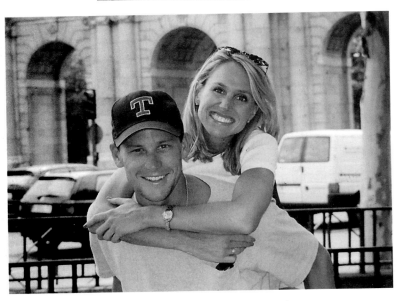

. . . and as a man in love. *(Courtesy of Kristin Armstrong)*

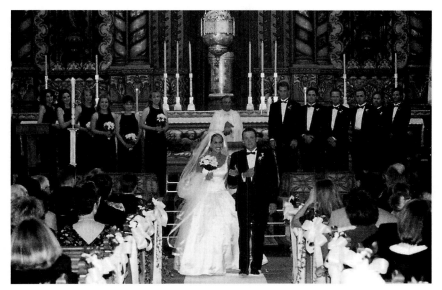

Our wedding day in Santa Barbara, followed by a great party. The bride and groom smoked cigars. *(Baron Spafford)*

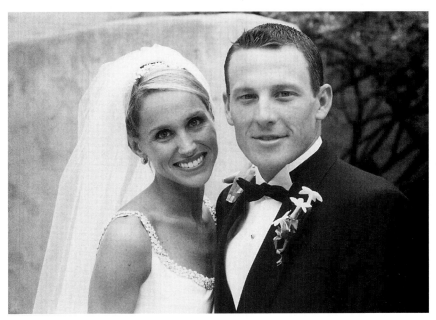

Mr. and Mrs. Lance Armstrong. I took the bike on our honeymoon. *(Baron Spafford)*

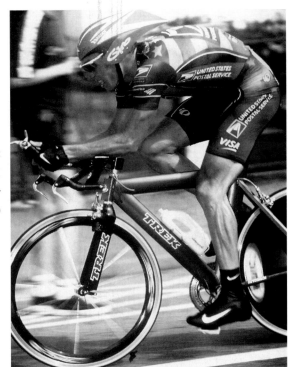

The Race of Truth: at
the time trial in Metz, I
took the yellow jersey for
good. *(Graham Watson)*

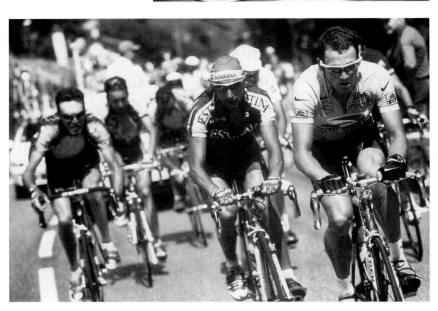

Stage 15: Controlling the mountains was key as I raced through the Pyrenees,
pursued by Fernando Escartin and Alex Zulle, on one of the toughest days of the
entire Tour. *(Graham Watson)*

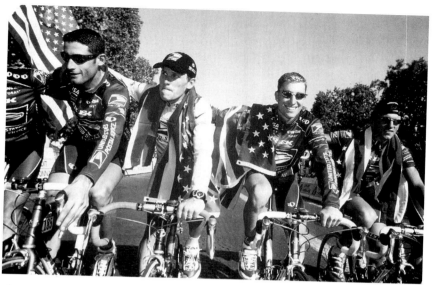

After three weeks and more than 2,387 miles, I shared the victory lap on the Champs-Elysées with my U.S. Postal teammates. *(James Startt)*

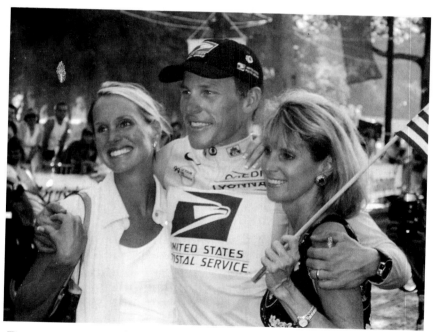

Reunited in Paris with Kik and my mom. *(Courtesy of Linda Armstrong)*

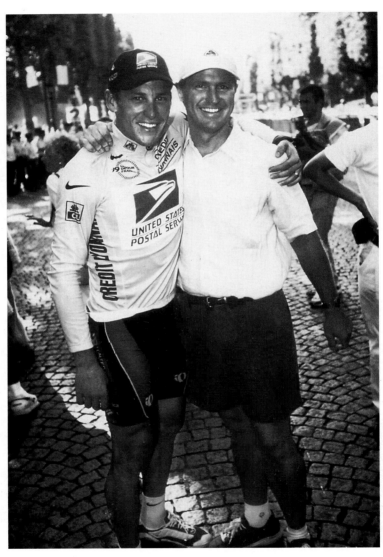

I proudly displayed the *maillot jaune* with my longtime friend
and coach, Chris Carmichael, who always told me
I would win it. *(James Startt)*

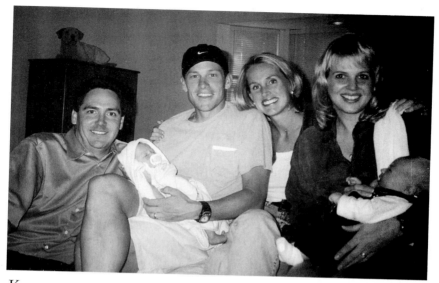

Kik and I with our friends Bill and Laura Stapleton, holding each other's children. Alex Stapleton was born just a few weeks after Luke. *(Colleen Capasso)*

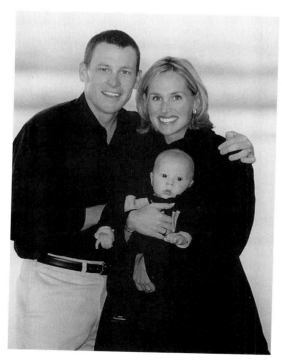

Luke David Armstrong with his parents. "My two miracle boys," Kik calls us. *(Baron Spafford)*

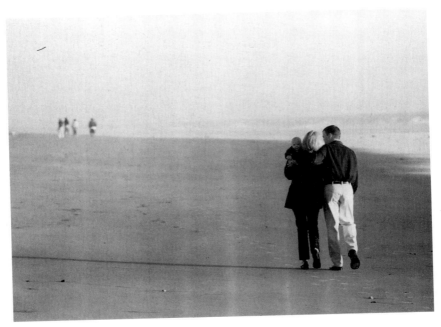

Walking into the sunset in Santa Barbara. *(Baron Spafford)*

get out of Plano, a potential source of wealth and recognition. But it was not something I did for pleasure, or poetry; it was my profession and my livelihood, and my reason for being, but I would not have said that I loved it.

I'd never ridden just to ride in the past—there had to be a purpose behind it, a race or a training regimen. Before, I wouldn't even consider riding for just thirty minutes or an hour. Real cyclists don't even take the bike out of the garage if it's only going to be an hour-long ride.

Bart would call up and say, "Let's go hang out and ride bikes."

"What for?" I'd say.

But now I not only loved the bike, I needed it. I needed to get away from my problems for a little while, and to make a point to myself and to my friends. I had a reason for those rides: I wanted everyone to see that I was okay, and still able to ride—and maybe I was trying to prove it to myself, too.

"How's Lance doing?" people would say.

I wanted my friends to say, "Well, he seems pretty good. He's riding his bike."

Maybe I needed to tell myself that I was still a rider, not just a cancer patient, no matter how weak I had become. If nothing else, it was my way of countering the disease and regaining the control it had stripped from me. *I can still do this,* I told myself. *I might not be able to do it like I used to, but I can still do it.*

Then one day Kevin and another friend and local cyclist, Jim Woodman, came over to take me for our usual little ride. I still had the scars from my surgery, so I wore a helmet, and we moved at a very slow pace, just idling along. Again, it wasn't anything I would have previously classified as a ride.

We came to a small rise in the road, nothing difficult at all, just an incline that required you to rise from your seat and stroke down on the pedals once or twice. I'd done it a million times. Up, down, and then sit and coast into a left-hand turn, and you're out of the neighborhood.

I couldn't do it. I got halfway up the incline, and I lost my breath. My bike wobbled beneath me, and I stopped, and put my feet down on the pavement. I felt faint.

I tried to breathe, but I couldn't seem to draw in enough air to revive myself. Black and silver specks fluttered behind my eyes. I dismounted. Kevin and Jim wheeled around and stopped short, concerned.

I sat down on the curb in front of a stranger's house and dropped my head between my knees.

Kevin was at my side in an instant. "Are you okay?" he said.

"Just let me catch my breath," I wheezed. "Go ahead without me, I'll get a ride home."

Jim said, "Maybe we should get an ambulance."

"No," I said. "Just let me sit here for a second."

I could hear myself trying to breathe. It sounded like *Whoo. Whoo.* Suddenly, even sitting up felt like too much effort. I felt a rushing light-headedness, similar to the sensation you get when you stand up too quickly—only I wasn't standing.

I lay back on the lawn, staring at the sky, and closed my eyes.

Is this dying?

Kevin hovered over me, distraught. "Lance!" he said, loudly. "Lance!"

I opened my eyes.

"I'm calling the ambulance," he said, desperately.

"No," I said, angrily. "No, no, I just need to rest."

"Okay, okay," he said, calming us both down.

After a few minutes, I gradually recovered my breath. I sat up, and tried to pull myself together. I stood. I tentatively straddled my bike.

My legs felt shaky, but I was able to ride downhill. We coasted very slowly back the way we came, and made our way back to my house. Kevin and Jim rode right next to me, never taking their eyes off me.

Between deep breaths, I explained to them what had happened. The chemo had robbed me of healthy blood cells and wiped out my hemoglobin count. Hemoglobin transports oxygen to your vital areas, and a normal value of hemoglobin for a fit person is about 13 to 15.

I was at seven. My blood was totally depleted. The chemo had attacked my blood relentlessly every two weeks, Monday through Friday, and I had finally overdone the bike riding.

I paid for it that day.

But I didn't stop riding.

THERE ARE ANGELS ON THIS EARTH AND THEY COME IN subtle forms, and I decided LaTrice Haney was one of them. Outwardly, she looked like just another efficient, clipboard-and-syringe-wielding nurse in a starched outfit. She worked extremely long days and nights, and on her off hours she went home to her husband, Randy, a truck driver, and their two children, Taylor, aged seven, and Morgan, four. But if she was tired, she never seemed it. She struck me as a woman utterly lacking in ordinary resentments, sure of her responsibilities and blessings and unwavering in her administering of care, and if that wasn't angelic behavior, I didn't know what was.

Often I'd be alone in the late afternoons and evenings except for LaTrice, and if I had the strength, we'd talk seriously. With most people I was shy and terse, but I found myself talking to LaTrice, maybe because she was so gentle-spoken and expressive herself. LaTrice was only in her late 20s, a pretty young woman with a coffee-and-cream complexion, but she had self-possession and perception beyond her years. While other people our age were out nightclubbing, she was already the head nurse for the oncology research unit. I wondered why she did it. "My satisfaction is to make it a little easier for people," she said.

She asked me about cycling, and I found myself telling her about the bike with a sense of pleasure I hadn't realized I possessed. "How did you start riding?" she asked me. I told her about my first bikes, and the early sense of liberation, and that cycling was all I had done since I was 16. I talked about my various teammates over the years, about their humor and selflessness, and I talked about my mother, and what she had meant to me.

I told her what cycling had given me, the tours of Europe and the extraordinary education, and the wealth. I showed her a picture of my house, with pride, and invited her to come visit, and I showed her snapshots of my cycling career. She leafed through images of me racing across the backdrops of France, Italy, and Spain, and she'd point to a picture and ask, "Where are you here?"

I confided that I was worried about my sponsor, Cofidis, and explained the difficulty I was having with them. I told her I felt pressured. "I need to stay in shape, I need to stay in shape," I said over and over again.

"Lance, listen to your body," she said gently. "I know your mind wants to run away. I know it's saying to you, 'Hey, let's go ride.' But listen to your body. Let it rest."

I described my bike, the elegant high performance of the ultralight tubing and aerodynamic wheels. I told her how much each piece cost, and weighed, and what its purpose was. I explained how a bike could be broken down so I could practically carry it in my pocket, and that I knew every part and bit of it so intimately that I could adjust it in a matter of moments.

I explained that a bike has to fit your body, and that at times I felt melded to it. The lighter the frame, the more responsive it is, and my racing bike weighed just 18 pounds. Wheels exert centrifugal force on the bike itself, I told her. The more centrifugal force, the more momentum. It was the essential building block of speed. "There are 32 spokes in a wheel," I said. Quick-release levers allow you to pop the wheel out and change it quickly, and my crew could fix a flat tire in less than 10 seconds.

"Don't you get tired of leaning over like that?" she asked.

Yes, I said, until my back ached like it was broken, but that was the price of speed. The handlebars are only as wide as the rider's shoulders, I explained, and they curve downward in half-moons so you can assume an aerodynamic stance on the bike.

"Why do you ride on those little seats?" she asked.

The seat is narrow, contoured to the anatomy, and the reason is that when you are on it for six hours at a time, you don't want anything to chafe your legs. Better a hard seat than the torture of saddle sores. Even the clothes have a purpose. They are flimsy for a reason: to mold to the body because you have to wear them in weather that ranges from hot to hail. Basically, they're a second skin. The shorts have a chamois padded seat, and the stitches are recessed to avoid rash.

When I had nothing left to tell LaTrice about the bike, I told her about the wind. I described how it felt in my face and in my hair. I told her about being in the open air, with the views of soaring Alps, and the glimmer of valley lakes in the distance. Sometimes the wind blew as if it were my personal friend, sometimes as if it were my bitter enemy, sometimes as if it were the hand of God pushing me along. I described the full sail of a mountain descent, gliding on two wheels only an inch wide.

"You're just out there, free," I said.

"You love it," she said.

"Yeah?" I said.

"Oh, I see it in your eyes," she said.

I understood that LaTrice was an angel one evening late in my last cycle of chemo. I lay on my side, dozing on and off, watching the steady, clear drip-drip of the chemo as it slid into my veins. LaTrice sat with me, keeping me company, even though I was barely able to talk.

"What do you think, LaTrice?" I asked, whispering. "Am I going to pull through this?"

"Yeah," she said. "Yeah, you are."

"I hope you're right," I said, and closed my eyes again.

LaTrice leaned over to me.

"Lance," she said, softly, "I hope someday to be just a figment of your imagination. I'm not here to be in your life for the rest of your life. After you leave here, I hope I never see you ever again. When you're cured, hey, let me see you in the papers, on TV, but not back here. I hope to help you at the time you need me, and then I hope I'll be gone. You'll say, 'Who was that nurse back in Indiana? Did I dream her?' "

It is one of the single loveliest things anyone has ever said to me. And I will always remember every blessed word.

ON DECEMBER 13, 1996, I TOOK MY LAST CHEMO treatment. It was almost time to go home.

Shortly before I received the final dose of VIP, Craig Nichols came by to see me. He wanted to talk with me about the larger implications of cancer. He wanted to talk about "the obligation of the cured."

It was a subject I had become deeply immersed in. I had said to Nichols and to LaTrice many times over the last three months, "People need to know about this." As I went through therapy, I felt increasing companionship with my fellow patients. Often I was too sick for much socializing, but one afternoon LaTrice asked me to go to the children's ward to talk to a young boy who was about to start his first cycle. He was scared and self-conscious, just like me. I visited with him for a while, and I told him, "I've been so sick. But I'm getting better." Then I showed him my driver's license.

In the midst of chemo, my license had expired. I could have put off renewing it until I felt better and had grown some hair back, but I decided not to. I pulled on some sweatclothes and hauled myself down to the Department of Motor Vehicles, and stood in front of the camera. I was completely bald, with no eyelashes or eyebrows, and my skin was the color of a pigeon's underbelly. But I looked into the lens, and I smiled.

"I wanted this picture so that when I got better, I would never forget how sick I've been," I said. "You *have* to fight."

After that, LaTrice asked me to speak with other patients more and more often. It seemed to help them to know that an athlete was fighting the fight alongside them. One afternoon LaTrice pointed out that I was still asking her questions, but the nature of them had changed. At first, the questions I had asked were strictly about myself, my own treatments, my doses, my particular problems. Now I asked about other people. I was startled to read that eight million Americans were living with some form of cancer; how could I possibly feel like mine was an isolated problem? "Can you believe how many people have this?" I asked LaTrice.

"You've changed," she said, approvingly. "You're going global."

Dr. Nichols told me that there was every sign now that I was going to be among the lucky ones who cheated the disease. He said that as my health improved, I might feel that I had a larger purpose than just myself. Cancer could be an opportunity as well as a responsibility. Dr. Nichols had seen all kinds of cancer patients become dedicated activists against the disease, and he hoped I would be one of them.

I hoped so, too. I was beginning to see cancer as something that I was given for the good of others. I wanted to launch a foundation, and

I asked Dr. Nichols for some suggestions about what it might accomplish. I wasn't yet clear on what the exact purpose of the organization would be; all I knew was that I felt I had a mission to serve others that I'd never had before, and I took it more seriously than anything in the world.

I had a new sense of purpose, and it had nothing to do with my recognition and exploits on a bike. Some people won't understand this, but I no longer felt that it was my role in life to be a cyclist. Maybe my role was to be a cancer survivor. My strongest connections and feelings were with people who were fighting cancer and asking the same question I was: "Am I going to die?"

I had talked to Steve Wolff about what I was feeling, and he said, "I think you were fated to get this type of illness. One, because maybe you could overcome it, and two, because your potential as a human was so much greater than just being a cyclist."

At the end of my third cycle of chemo, I had called Bill Stapleton and said, "Can you research what it takes to start a charitable foundation?" Bill and Bart and another close friend and amateur cyclist, John Korioth, met with me one afternoon at an Austin restaurant to kick around some ideas. We had no idea how to go about launching a foundation, or how to raise money, but by the end of the lunch we came up with the idea of staging a charity bicycle race around Austin. We would call it the Ride for the Roses. I asked if anyone would have time to oversee the project, and Korioth raised his hand. Korioth was a bartender at a nightspot where I had hung out some in my former life, and I would even take a turn as a guest bartender occasionally. He said his schedule would allow him to put some real time into it. It was the perfect solution: we didn't want a lot of overhead, and whatever we raised, we wanted to give straight back to the cause.

But I still wasn't clear on the basic purpose of the foundation. I knew that because my case was such a *cause célèbre* people would listen, but I didn't want the foundation as a pulpit for me personally. I didn't think I was special—and I would never know how much a part of my own cure I was. On the meaning of it, I wasn't really clear. All I wanted to do was tell people, "Fight like hell, just like I did."

As I talked to Dr. Nichols about how I could help, I decided that I wanted the foundation to involve research. I was so indebted to Dr. Einhorn and Dr. Nichols for their erudition, I wanted to try to pay them back in some small way for all of the energy and caring that they and their staff had put into my well-being. I envisioned a scientific advisory board that would review requests for funding and decide which ones were the best and most worthy, and dole the money out accordingly.

But there were so many fronts to the cancer fight that I couldn't focus solely on one. I had a host of new friends who were involved in the fight, directly and indirectly, patients, doctors, nurses, families, and scientists, and I was beginning to feel closer to them than to some cyclists I knew. The foundation could keep me tied very closely to all of them.

I wanted the foundation to manifest all of the issues I had dealt with in the past few months: coping with fear, the importance of alternate opinions, thorough knowledge of the disease, the patient's role in cure, and above all, the idea that cancer did not have to be a death sentence. It could be a route to a second life, an inner life, a better life.

AFTER THE FINAL CHEMO TREATMENT, I STAYED IN THE hospital for a couple more days, recovering my strength and tying up loose ends. One of the loose ends was my catheter. The day that it was removed was a momentous occasion for me, because I had been living with it for nearly four months. I said to Nichols, "Hey, can we take this thing out?"

He said, "Sure."

I felt a surge of relief—if he agreed to take it out, he must have been confident I wouldn't need it again. No more chemo, hopefully.

The next day an intern came to my room and removed that ugly, torturous device from my chest. But there were complications; the thing had been buried in me for so long that it had grown into my skin. The intern dug around, and couldn't get it out. He had to call in a more experienced doctor, who practically ripped it out of my chest. It was agony. I even imagined I heard a tearing noise as it came out. Next, the gash it left became infected and they had to go back in and perform a day surgery to clean out the wound and sew me up again. It was awful, maybe the worst experience of the whole four months, and I was so mad when it was finally over that I demanded the catheter. I wanted to keep it, and I still have it, in a little Ziploc bag, a memento.

There was one more detail to discuss: Nichols gave me a final analysis of my health. I would have to go through a period of uncertainty. Quite often the final chemo treatment did not erase every trace of cancer, and I would need monthly blood tests and checkups to ensure that the disease was in full retreat. He warned me that my blood markers were not quite normal and my chest X ray still showed signs of scar tissue from the tumors.

I was concerned. Nichols said, reassuringly, "We see it a lot. These are minor abnormalities, and we're highly confident they will go away." If I was cured, the scar tissue and markers should resolve themselves in time. But there was no guarantee; the first year was key. If the disease was going to come back, that's when we would see it.

I wanted to be cured, and cured now. I didn't want to wait a year to find out.

I went back home, and tried to piece my life back together. I took it easy at first, just played a little golf and worked on plans for the foundation. As my system cleaned out, my body didn't seem broken by the chemo, I realized with relief. But I still felt like a cancer patient, and the feelings I'd held at bay for the last three months began to surface.

One afternoon I agreed to play a little golf with Bill Stapleton and another friend of ours named Dru Dunworth, who was a lymphoma survivor, at a club called Onion Creek. My hair hadn't grown back yet, and I wasn't supposed to get a lot of sun, so I put on one of those goofy caps that you pull down over your ears. I went into the pro shop to buy some balls. There was a young guy working behind the counter. He looked at me, smirking, and said, "Are you going to wear that hat?"

"Yeah," I said shortly.

"Don't you think it's warm out there?" he said.

I ripped the hat off so he could see that I was bald and scarred, and leaped across the counter.

"You see these fucking scars?" I snarled.

The guy backed away.

"That's why I'm going to wear that hat," I said. "Because I have cancer."

I pulled the cap on and I stalked out of the shop, so angry I was trembling.

I was tense, admittedly. I still spent a lot of time at the doctor's offices. I had blood drawn each week by Dr. Youman so the doctors in Indianapolis could keep track of me. I was constantly monitored. With an illness like cancer, monitoring is critical, and you live by the results, the blood work, CT scans, MRIs. You live by knowing your progress. In my case, I'd had a fast-growing cancer that had gone away quickly—but it could come back just as quickly.

One day after I had been back in Austin for a few weeks, LaTrice called Dr. Youman for the numbers. After she wrote them down, she took them to Dr. Nichols. He looked at the sheet of paper she had handed him, and he smiled and gave it back to her. "Why don't you call him this time," he said.

LaTrice dialed my home phone. Like I say, the numbers were all-important for me, and I would wait nervously by the phone for every result. I picked up right away.

"We got the blood counts back," LaTrice said.

"Yeah?" I said, nervously.

"Lance, they're normal," she said.

I held the thought up in my mind and looked at it: I was no longer sick. I might not stay that way; I still had a long year ahead of me, and if the illness returned it would probably happen in the next 12 months. But for this moment, at least for this brief and priceless moment, there wasn't a physical trace of cancer left in my body.

I didn't know what to say. I was afraid if I opened my mouth, nothing would come out but one long, inarticulate shout of relief.

"I'm so glad I can bring you good news," LaTrice said.

I sighed.

seven

KIK

LOVE AND CANCER WERE STRANGE COMPAN-
ions, but in my case they came along at the same time. It was hardly
the ideal situation in which to meet my future wife—but that's exactly
what happened. Why do two people get married? For a future together, naturally. The question was whether or not I had one.

I didn't have cancer anymore, but I didn't *not* have it, either. I was
in a state of anxiety called remission, and I was obsessed with the idea
of a relapse. I would wake up in the night with phantom pains in my
chest, and I'd lie in bed in the darkness, covered in sweat and listening
to the sound of my own breathing, convinced the tumors had come
back. The next morning I'd go directly to the doctor and ask for a
chest X ray to calm myself down.

"The chemo works or it doesn't," Dr. Einhorn once said. "If it works, the patient lives a normal, cancer-free life. If it doesn't and the cancer comes back, he will usually be dead in three or four months." It was that simple.

Getting on with my life, on the other hand, was much more complicated. I finished chemotherapy on December 13, 1996, and I met Kristin Richard a month later, at a press conference to announce the launching of my cancer foundation and the Ride for the Roses. We spoke just briefly. She was a slim blond woman who everyone called Kik (pronounced Keek), an account executive for an advertising and public-relations firm in town, assigned to help promote the event. I know I'm supposed to say the light changed when I saw her, but actually, it didn't. I just thought she was smart and pretty. She told me later her first impression of me was equally inconsequential. I was "a cute bald guy with a great smile." It would be spring before we had deeper feelings, and summer before we acted on them. For one thing, we were seeing other people, and for another, the first time we ever talked at length we had a fight.

It started on the phone. She represented a corporate client, a major title sponsor of the Ride for the Roses, and she felt I wasn't doing enough to please them. One afternoon she got testy with a foundation staffer. *Who is this chick?* I thought, and dialed her number, and as soon as she answered I said, "This is Lance Armstrong, and what do you mean by talking to my staff that way?" I went off, barking at her. On the other end of the receiver, Kik rolled her eyes, thinking, *This guy acts like he is so big-time.*

For the next ten minutes we argued back and forth.

"Obviously, this conversation is going nowhere," she snapped.

"Damn right it's going nowhere!" I snapped back.

"You know what?" she said. "We need to talk about this over a beer. That's all I have to say to you."

I was nonplussed. "Oh, uh, okay. We'll go have a beer."

I invited her to meet up with me and a couple of friends at a local bar. I don't think either of us expected to be as drawn to the other as we were. I was still pale and washed out and fatigued from the illness, but she didn't seem to care. She was funnier and more easygoing than I had anticipated, and very bright. I asked her to join the weekly foundation meetings at my house, and she agreed.

The foundation seemed like the perfect answer to the limbo I was in: I had completed chemo, and beaten back the cancer for the time being, but I had to figure out what to do next. To work on something outside myself was the best antidote. I was a cancer survivor first and an athlete second, I decided. Too many athletes live as though the problems of the world don't concern them. We are isolated by our wealth and our narrow focus, and our elitism. But one of the redeeming things about being an athlete—one of the real services we can perform—is to redefine what's humanly possible. We cause people to reconsider their limits, to see that what looks like a wall may really just be an obstacle in the mind. Illness was not unlike athletic performance in that respect: there is so much we don't know about our human capacity, and I felt it was important to spread the message.

One of the more important events of that winter–spring was that I met a man named Jeff Garvey, a prominent Austin venture capitalist who would become a close friend in time, but who at first I simply hoped would help guide the foundation. A mutual acquaintance introduced us, and Jeff invited me to lunch. I drove up to his place in my Explorer in shorts and a T-shirt. We had a long rambling lunch, and talked about cycling—Jeff was an avid amateur rider and each year he made a trip through Spain, following the famous Camino de Santiago. Jeff had lost both of his parents to cancer, and he was looking for some charitable work to do in fighting the disease. A few weeks later, I asked Jeff to have lunch with me again, and over the meal I asked him if he would take over the running of the foundation. He agreed, and became our CEO.

For the next two months Kik and I worked together on the foundation. At first, she just seemed like a stylish girl who always had a quick comeback. Gradually, though, I found myself noticing her long fine blond hair, and the way she would make the most casual clothes look classy somehow. And then there was her Colgate commercial of a smile. It was hard not to get lost in the view. Also, I liked her sass. Meanwhile, Kik had started reading up on me in her spare time, under the pretext of doing research for business purposes. But neither of us was willing to admit how we felt yet.

We held the inaugural Ride for the Roses in March, and it was a big success. We raised over $200,000, and the Wallflowers played a concert, and friends and colleagues came from all over the world to ride, including Miguel Indurain, Eddy Merckx, and Eric Heiden.

There was one donation I'll never forget. I was sitting at a table doing an autograph signing, with a huge line stretching down the block, scribbling my name as fast as possible. I signed over and over, barely glancing upward as each person stepped in front of me.

A checkbook flew in my face and flopped open on the table.

"How much do you want?" a voice said.

Without looking up, I said, "Goddamn."

I started to laugh and shake my head. I knew that voice. It was the long-lost Jim Hoyt, my homeboy from Plano, the man who put me on my first bike and then took my beloved Camaro away. He was standing right in front of me, and so was his wife, Rhonda. I hadn't laid eyes on them since our bitter disagreement a decade earlier. I looked Jim in the eye.

"I'm sorry," I said. I figured I owed him that.

"Accepted," he said. "Now, how much do I make it out for?"

"Jim, you don't have to do that."

"No," he said. "I want to help."

"Aw, come on, don't do this," I said.

"How about five grand? Does that sound good?"

I burst out laughing. Five grand was what I had put into that Camaro. "That'd be fine," I said.

He wrote out the check, and we shook hands.

Every year, Jim always comes back for the Ride. And I mean to tell you, homeboy goes crazy with his checkbook, and he never asks me for a thing in return.

A little while later, another memorable person stepped in front of me: a little girl whose head was semi-bald like mine. Our eyes met, and we connected instantly. As I signed an autograph for her, she recited all of my stats: she knew everything about my career. Her name was Kelly Davidson and she was a cancer patient, and for days afterward I couldn't get her out of my mind. I tracked her down and called her, and we became good friends.

I SHOULD HAVE KNOWN I WAS IN TROUBLE WITH KIK when we kept thinking up reasons to see each other after the Ride was over. We would exchange e-mails a lot, and talk on the phone, and find excuses to meet now and then beyond foundation meetings. She continued to come to the weekly gatherings at my house, and one night she stayed after everybody else left. It was just the two of us, sitting in my living room sipping beers and talking. I remember thinking, *What am I doing? Why am I here alone with her?* She was thinking the exact same thing. Finally, she stood up to call a cab, and I offered to give her a ride home.

We drove through the empty dark streets, not saying much of anything, but feeling a lot. There was something there, but neither of us was ready to touch it yet. So we just drove.

BY SPRING OF '97, I WASN'T EXACTLY READY TO GO
out for margaritas. The medical uncertainties were still a constant,
nagging worry. "What's it going to be?" I'd ask Dr. Nichols. "Am I
going to live or die? What?"

I felt pressure to get back on my bike, and yet I was unsure of my
body. I counted and recounted my financial assets and sweated every
mortgage payment, wondering if I would ever make another dime
from cycling. Finally, I decided to at least try to race; I could still lock
Cofidis into the second year of the contract and relieve myself of financial worries if I appeared in four events. I told Bill, "Let's find
some races."

A month after leaving the hospital, I'd flown to France to appear at
a Cofidis press conference. The team officials were shocked that I
showed up, but I wanted them to see that I was not the pale, bedrid-
den victim they had left in Indianapolis. I told the Cofidis people that
I wanted to try to come back in the spring, and I even spent a couple
of days riding and working out with the team. They seemed pleased.

I began to train seriously, riding four hours a day, as much as 100
miles over some of the old routes I used to love, ranging from Austin
to Wimberly, to Dripping Springs, to New Sweden, towns with nothing but cotton fields and tractors and solitary church steeples in the distance. But I didn't like how I was feeling. Sometimes I would ride for
an hour or so, just a little cruise, and it wore me out and I'd have to
take a long nap afterward. I rode at a moderate pace, only about 130
heartbeats per minute, but I would feel strong one day and weak the
next.

I had a vague, run-down sensation that was all too familiar: it was
the way I had felt before the diagnosis, I realized, with a knot in my
stomach. Then I got a cold. I was sleepless and paralyzed with fear for

an entire night, certain the cancer had come back. Before the illness I had never been susceptible to colds; if I was coming down with something, it had to be cancer.

The next morning I raced to see Dr. Youman for a checkup, certain he would tell me I was ill again. But it was just a common infection that my body wasn't strong enough to fight off. My immune system was shot, and I was what the doctors called "neutrophilic": my white blood cell count was still down, which meant I was susceptible to every little germ that came along.

My X rays had not entirely cleared up, either. There was a spot of some kind in my abdomen. The doctors didn't know quite what it was, and decided just to keep an eye on it. I was a nervous wreck.

That was it. Dr. Nichols recommended that I take the rest of the year off, and I agreed; there would be no serious cycling for me in '97. I was still convalescing, Nichols explained, and my immune system hadn't fully rebounded from a chemo regimen that had been far more strenuous than I realized. My lack of fitness was in no way related to lack of will, Nichols said, it was a simple matter of how much the illness had taken out of me.

My friends and colleagues felt like I did, nervous. "Look," Och said. "Whatever you decide, make sure the doctors know exactly what you're doing, training-wise, how much you're working. Give them the details so they can make the determination as to how hard you should go."

I had to admit it: I might never legitimately race again at the top level. Maybe my body just couldn't deal with the rigors of a full-time training regimen.

Chris Carmichael called me and wanted to know what was going on.

"Chris, I'm scared," I said. "I'm scared to train. I'm scared if I push myself too hard, it will come back."

———————

IN AN ODD WAY, HAVING CANCER WAS EASIER THAN RE-covery—at least in chemo I was *doing* something, instead of just waiting for it to come back.

Some days I still called myself a bike racer, and some days I didn't. One afternoon I went to play golf with Bill at a local country club. We were on the fifth hole, a par-5, and Bill hit a beautiful six-iron for a chance at eagle. "I'll be able to do that some day," I said, admiringly.

Bill said, "It's going to be a while before you play enough golf to hit a shot like that."

"Bill, you don't get it," I said. "I'm retired."

Bill and I had this argument all the time. I vacillated—one day I would plan my big comeback, and the next day I would tell him my career was over.

On the first tee, I'd say, "Well, now we're just friends because I don't need an agent anymore. I'm never riding again." A few minutes later I'd be standing on the next tee, waggling a club, and I'd say, "When I start riding again, what are we going to do, what's the plan?" By the next hole, I would have reversed myself again.

"I hope you're not hanging out with me because you think I'm going to make any more money," I'd say. "Because I'm not riding."

Bill knew I was prone to making sweeping statements, and he had learned to make a joke, or to put me off. He'd say to me, "Okay, fine, we'll talk about this tomorrow."

Then something happened that deepened my ambivalence: Bill's assistant, our good friend Stacy Pounds, was diagnosed with lung cancer. Stacy had been a tremendous help to me during my own illness and an integral partner in launching the foundation. She was a 55-year-old Texas belle and chain-smoker, with a gritty voice and exquisite manners. Stacy could basically tell you that you were the biggest jerk in the world, and to never call again, and that you smelled, too, but you would hang up thinking, "That was the nicest lady."

Stacy was not as fortunate as I was; her cancer was incurable. We were devastated, and all we could do was try to support her and make her more comfortable. My mother came across two pretty silver crucifixes on chains, and bought them for me. I wore one, and I gave the other to Stacy. She was completely agnostic, just like me, but I said, "Stacy, I want to give you this cross, and I'm going to wear one, too. This is going to be our bond. You wear it when you're being treated, or wear it whenever you want. And I'll wear mine forever." We wore them not as religious symbols but universal ones, symbols of our cancer kinship.

Stacy deteriorated quickly. One day she announced, "I'm not doing chemotherapy if I can't get better." Dr. Youman tried to treat her, but the chemo wasn't working. It made her miserably sick, and it wasn't going to save her life, either. Ultimately, she stopped, and the doctor told us she had only a matter of weeks left.

Stacy had a son, Paul, who was a sailor serving with the Navy at sea, and we wanted to bring him home to see his mother, but nobody seemed able to get him off his ship. We called congressmen and senators, everybody, but nothing happened. Finally I decided to pull a string; I knew a four-star general, Charles Boyd, who'd been based in Germany, and who had recently retired and was living in Washington. I dialed his number, and I said, "General Boyd, I need a favor."

I explained about Stacy, and I said, "This lady's dying, and her son's on board a ship." General Boyd stopped me. "Lance," he said, "you don't need to say any more. I lost my wife two years ago to cancer. I'll see what I can do." The next day, the kid was on his way home. That's what the term "cancer community" means.

But before Paul got home, Stacy went into a nursing home for a few days. A group of us went to visit her there, Bill, me, and my mom, and we found her in an awful, crowded facility with barely enough nurses to go around. Stacy said, "I'm in pain. I ring the bell in the night and they don't bring me my pain medicine." I was horrified.

I said, "Stacy, this is the deal. We're going to pack up your shit, and we're going to check you out of here. You're going to go home, and I'm going to hire you a full-time nurse."

A nursing-home official said, "You can't check her out."

"She's fucking leaving," I said. "Now."

I told Bill, "Back the car up. Open the door." And we were gone. Stacy spent her last few weeks at home. Her son arrived, and we found a hospice nurse to help him care for her. She fought as hard as she could, and held out for three weeks more than the doctors predicted. She was diagnosed in January, right after I finished my own chemo. She quit working in February, and by March she was gravely ill. Then she slipped away, and broke all our hearts.

I was despondent, and still nervous about my own health, and half guilty over my good fortune in being alive. Cycling didn't seem like a very important pursuit after losing Stacy, and I didn't think it was a realistic one, either. Steve Lewis came from Plano for a visit, and could see an obvious change in me. I don't think he understood what the illness had done to me until he laid eyes on me, so skinny and white, cheekbones sticking out, and defeated-seeming. I showed Steve the pictures of my lungs, and I told him, "I really thought I was going to die."

I was still struggling to get past the idea that I could have lost my life, and it was difficult to know where to begin again. Decisions like whether to try to race, and how to deal with Cofidis, were beyond me. I didn't know what I wanted, or even what was possible, and I couldn't help feeling that cycling was trivial.

Steve looked at a picture of me winning a stage of the Tour de France, and he said, "When are you going to do this again?"

"I'm pretty sure I'm done with that," I said. "It's too hard on your body."

"You're kidding," Steve said, shocked.

"I'll never be able to ride in that race again," I said.

Steve was taken aback. He had never known me to give up at anything. "I think I've lost it," I said. "I just don't feel good on the bike." I told him I was afraid of losing my house, and that I had tried to adjust to certain spending restrictions. I had scaled things back proportionately, and tried to come up with an alternate plan for the future, with no bikes in it. Steve knew me as a braggadocious kid, but now I was talking like a victim. I didn't have the edge that he remembered.

As for my personal life, I was equally tentative. Lisa and I needed to make some decisions about our future together, and I had seriously considered marriage. She had stayed with me throughout the cancer battle, every miserable step of the way, and that meant something. She gave me a kitten, and we named it Chemo.

"I think she's the one," I'd told Steve. "She stuck with me through this, and she'll stick with me through anything."

But when Steve came back to see me again two months later, Lisa and I had broken up. That tells you how chaotic my feelings were. Cancer does one of two things to a relationship: it either brings you closer together, or it tears you apart. In our case, it tore us apart. As I began to slowly recover, we found that we had less and less to talk about. Maybe it was just a case of exhaustion; we had spent so much energy fighting the illness and gotten through all of the hard parts, but in the end it left us numb, too. One day in March, she said, "Let's see other people."

"Okay," I said.

But soon we were hardly seeing each other at all. Lisa certainly understood that I had been sick—but it was harder for her to understand why I didn't have any emotional wherewithal left. We continued to see each other on and off—you don't just completely sever a relationship like that. But it ended, just the same.

I was so confused about what to do with myself that one afternoon I went for a bike ride with Bill (ordinarily, I would never ride with such a novice), and as we pedaled slowly around my neighborhood, I said, "I'm going back to college to be an oncologist. Or maybe I'll go to business school."

Bill just shook his head. He had a master's degree in business, and a law degree from the University of Texas as well. "You know, I went to college for eleven years," Bill said. "I had to sweat it out in school, and I'll have to sweat it the rest of my life. You don't ever have to do that, dude. Why do you want to go to work every day on a trading floor at four-thirty in the morning, if you don't have to?"

"You don't get it, Bill," I said. "I keep telling you, I'm not a biker now."

For a while, Kik stopped calling me back; I couldn't reach her no matter how hard I tried. She was unsure about me, because she had heard about my reputation as a player, and she didn't intend to be a casualty. I wasn't used to being cut dead, and it drove me crazy. I left message after message on her machine. "Are you ever going to call me back?" I demanded.

Finally, Kik relented. I didn't know it, but her life was in transition, too. She split with the man she had been seeing, and she changed jobs, all within a few weeks. Finally, one afternoon she answered her phone when I called.

I said, "Well, what's new?"

"A lot. I just started this new job, and I'm busy."

"Oh," I said. Then I took a deep breath. "Damn. I thought you were going to tell me that you were single."

"Well, funny you should mention it. I am. I broke up two days ago."

"Really?" I said, trying to sound casual. "You're single?"

"Yeah."

"So what are you doing tonight?" I asked.

"Something with you," she said.

We've been together ever since.

I knew instantly I had met my match. Kik could handle herself; she was tough, independent, sensible, and unspoiled. Although she had grown up around money—her father was an executive of a Fortune 500 company—she was used to taking care of herself and didn't expect anything to be handed to her. *I think I get it now,* I thought to myself.

I felt safe with her. She liked me bald and sick with no eyebrows, and the insecurities I might have had about my hair, my scars, my body, didn't seem to matter. Kik became my hairstylist. She would take my head in her hands and gently trim my hair with a pair of clippers until I looked like a 1960s astronaut.

I'd always had the upper hand in my relationships, but not with Kik. Sometimes I would lead, and sometimes I would follow, but mostly I would go where she wanted me to go. Still do. North, south, east, and all the rest. That summer, Kik had plans to go to Europe. She had never been overseas, and a friend of hers from college, an exchange student who lived in Spain, wanted her to come visit. "Why are you going to Spain?" I said. "Spain's a dustbowl."

"Shut up," Kik said. "Don't ruin my fun, I've been saving for this for years."

She would be gone for over a month. That was totally unacceptable, I decided. There was only one thing to do: go with her. I was supposed to make an appearance at the Tour de France, as a courtesy to my sponsors and to show that I was still a potentially viable competitor, and I decided to time it with Kik's trip. I was curious to see the Tour from a spectator's point of view, anyway, and I hoped it would revive my desire to cycle. I asked to go with her, and she agreed.

It was an awakening. I felt like I had never seen Europe before, and the truth is, maybe I hadn't. I had seen it from a bike, at 40 miles an hour, but I hadn't seen it as a tourist, and I hadn't seen it in love. We went everywhere. I showed off my French, my Italian, and my Spanish.

I had missed most of my 20s. I was too busy being a pro athlete and making a living from the age of 15 on to do the things most people in their 20s do, to have fun the way Kik and her college friends had fun. I'd completely skipped that phase of my life, but now I had a chance to go back and live it. I was still tentative about what would happen to my health, not knowing what I had left, if it was just one day, or two years, or a long life. *Carpe diem,* I told myself, seize the day. Whatever I had, I was going to spend it well. And that's how Kik and I found each other.

I had never embraced my life. I had made something of it, and fought for it, but I had never particularly enjoyed it. "You have this gift," Kik said. "You can teach me how to really love life, because you've been on the brink, and you saw the other side. So you can show me that."

But she showed me. She wanted to see everything, and I was the guy who got to show it to her, and in showing it to her, I saw it for myself. In Italy, we sat at sidewalk cafés and ate ham with shaved Parmesan cheese. Kik teased me, "Before I met you, Parmesan came in a green can."

We went to San Sebastián, where it had rained so hard that it hurt and the crowds had laughed at me as I finished last in my first pro race. This time, I gazed at the tiled roofs and the steppes of the city along the Bay of Biscay and decided that, contrary to my dismissive statement about dustbowls, there was nothing more beautifully old than Spain.

In Pamplona we saw the running of the bulls. Kik said, "Let's stay up all night long."

I said, "Why?"

"For fun. You mean you've never stayed up all night, and walked home in the sunrise?"

"No," I said.

"What do you *mean,* you've never stayed up all night?" she said. "That's *insane.* What's *wrong* with you?"

We stayed up all night. We went to every nightspot and dance club in Pamplona, and then we walked back to the hotel as the sun came up and lighted the gray plinth streets until they turned gold. Kik seemed to think I was sensitive and romantic—although few of my friends would have believed it. Chris Carmichael had always described me "kind of like an iceberg. There's a peak, but there's so much more below the surface." Kik was certain of it.

In Monaco, I told her that I loved her.

We were dressing for dinner in our hotel room, when suddenly we both grew quiet. Up to that moment, it had all been undercurrents. But as I watched her from across the room, I knew exactly what I was feeling, the tangled twisted strands of love. Only Kik was clear to me. Other than her, I was living in a state of utter confusion; I didn't know if I was going to live or die, and if I did live, I had no idea what I would do with my life. I didn't know what I wanted out of cycling anymore. I didn't know whether I wanted to ride, or retire, or go to college, or become a stockbroker. But I loved Kik.

"I think I'm in love with you," I said from across the room.

Kik stopped in the mirror and said, "You think you are? Or you know? Because I need to know. I really need to know."

"I know."

"I know it too," she said.

If you could ever hope to meet someone and fall in love, it should happen just as it did for us, blissfully, perfectly. Our relationship tended to be unspoken, a matter of a lot of deep, intense gazing, and a complex strum of emotions. The funny thing is, we never discussed my cancer—the only time we talked about it was when we talked about children. I told her that I did want them, and about the trip to San Antonio.

But it was frightening for us, too. Kik used to say, "I would never do anything for a man. I would never change my life just for a guy." She was like me, always in control of her relationships, emotions in check, independent, never the one to get hurt, didn't want anything from anyone, too tough for that. But by now our guards were totally down. One night, she admitted it to me. "If you want to just annihilate me, you can," she said. "Because there's nothing left to block you. So be careful what you do."

We went to the Tour de France. I tried to describe the race to her; the chess match among riders and the ten million fans lining the roads, but when she saw the peloton for herself, the palette of colors streaking by with the Pyrenees looming in the background, she screamed with joy.

I had business to do at the Tour, sponsors to see and reporters to talk to. By then I was so caught up in Kik and enjoying my second life that I sounded ambivalent about ever riding again.

"I'm just not as competitive as before," I told reporters. "Maybe I'm just a recreational cyclist now." Even though I was back on my bike, I told them, "I'm a participant, not a competitor." The Tour, I said, "is most likely impossible."

"Look," I said. "Cycling for me was really a job. It was very good to me. I did it for five or six years, lived all over Europe, did all the traveling. Now I have time to spend with my friends and family, do the stuff I missed doing my entire childhood."

BY THE END OF THE SUMMER I RESEMBLED A HEALTHY
person. I no longer looked sick, and I had all of my hair. But I still worried constantly about a relapse, and I had continuing ghost pains in my
chest.

I had nightmares. I had strange physical reactions; for no apparent
reason I would break out in a sweat. The slightest stress or anxiety
would cause my body to become shiny with perspiration.

While I was being treated I was actively killing the cancer, but
when the treatment stopped, I felt powerless, like I wasn't doing anything but waiting for the other shoe to fall. I was such an active, aggressive person that I would have felt better if they'd given me chemo
for a year. Dr. Nichols tried to reassure me. "Some people have more
trouble after treatment than during. It's common. It's more difficult to
wait for it to come back than it is to attack it."

The monthly checkups were the worst. Kik and I would fly to Indianapolis and check into the hotel adjacent to the medical center. The
next day I would rise at 5 A.M. to drink a contrast dye for the various
MRIs and scans and X rays, nasty stuff that tasted like a combination
of Tang and liquid metal. It was a grim experience to wake up in that
hotel again, and to know that I would have to sit in another doctor's
office and perhaps hear the words *You have cancer.*

Kik would wake up and sit with me as I choked down the cocktail of dye, slumped over and miserable. She would rub my back while
I swallowed it down. Once, to make me feel better, she even asked to
taste it. She took a swig and made a face. Like I say, she's a stud.

Then we'd walk over to the hospital to face the blood tests and the
MRIs. The doctors would line the chest X rays up on the light box
and flip the switch, and I would duck my head, afraid that I would see

those white spots again. Kik didn't know how to read an X ray, and the tension was racking for both of us. Once, she pointed at something and said, nervously, "What's this?"

"That's a rib," I said.

As we sat there, we both thought the same thing: *I've finally found the love of my life, the person who means everything in the world to me, and if anything takes that away now I will come unglued.* It was a sickening sensation then, and it's still sickening now, just to think about it.

But each X ray was clear, and the blood tests remained normal. With every passing month the chances of a relapse lessened.

I was no longer strictly convalescing. For all intents and purposes, I was healthy. As the one-year mark approached, Chris Carmichael began to urge me to race again. Finally, he flew to Austin to have it out with me. He believed I needed to get on my bike in earnest, that I had some unfinished business in the sport and that I was starting to seem empty without it, and he wasn't afraid to say so, either.

Chris had a long conversation with Bill Stapleton and said, "Everyone tells him to do what he wants, and no one will talk to him about racing his bike." He thought I needed a push, and our relationship had always been based on his ability to give me one when I needed it.

I knew exactly why Chris had come to see me. I told John Korioth, "Carmichael is in town to try to get me to race again, and I don't know if I want to." Chris and I went out to lunch at my favorite Tex-Mex place, Chuy's, and my prediction was correct.

"Lance," Chris said, "what is with this playing golf? Cycling is what you're about."

I shook my head skeptically. "I don't know," I said.

"Are you afraid?"

I was. I had been strong as a bull on the bike, and what if I wasn't anymore? Or what if racing could make me sick again?

"None of your doctors will say that you can race again," Chris said. "But none of them will say that you *can't,* either. I think you should try it, give it a run. I know it's a big unknown, a big risk, a big challenge, and a big scare. There are no givens. But here you are, back to life, and now you need to get back to living."

I thought it over for a couple of days. It's one thing to undergo chemo and go back to work as an accountant. But to be a cyclist? I didn't know about that. Chemo had made the worst climb in the Alps seem flat.

There was another factor to consider: I had a disability policy that would pay for five years. But if I made a comeback, I would forfeit the policy. I would be jumping off a financial cliff to race again.

Chris hung out and met Kik, and continued to badger me about getting back on the bike. I explained to him that I just wasn't clear on what I was supposed to do with the rest of my life, but he refused to believe it. At one point, he turned to Kik, and said, "Do *you* think he should race again?

"I don't really care," she said. "I'm in love with this man."

Chris looked at me. "Okay," he said. "You can marry her."

FINALLY, I MADE MY MIND UP: I WOULD TRY TO RACE again. I got back on the bike, and this time, I felt good about it. I told Bill and Kik, "I think I can do this." I asked Chris to formulate a training program for me, and I began to ride hard. But oddly enough, my body refused to take its previous shape. The old me had weighed 175 pounds. Now I was 158, my face looked narrow and hawkish, and you could see every sinew in my legs.

Bill called Cofidis and told them I was up and riding. "I want to talk to you about his racing program; he's ready to make a comeback," Bill said. The Cofidis people suggested that Bill come to France for a meeting.

Bill flew to Paris overnight, and then drove four hours into the country to reach the Cofidis executive offices. He arrived in time for an elegant lunch. Among those at the table were Alain Bondue and the Cofidis executive officer, François Migraine.

Migraine gave a five-minute speech, welcoming Bill to France. And then he said, "We want to thank you for coming here, but we want you to know that we're going to exercise our right to terminate his contract. We need to go in a different direction."

Bill looked at Bondue and said, "Is he serious?"

Bondue looked down at his plate and simply said, "Yes."

"Is there a reason I had to fly all the way over here for you to tell me that?" Bill asked.

"We thought it was important that we tell you person-to-person," Bondue said.

"Look, you only have to pay him a minimal amount to ride," Bill said. "Just let him race. He really wants to make a comeback. It's serious. It's not that we think he'll ride, we know he will."

Cofidis wasn't confident that I would ever ride at that level again, and what's more, if I did ride, and I happened to get sick again, it would be bad publicity for Cofidis.

It was over. Bill was desperate. "Look, he's been part of your team; you paid him. At least make us an offer." Finally, the Cofidis people said they would consider it.

Bill left without finishing lunch, and got back in his car for the long drive back to Paris. He couldn't stand to break the news to me, and he drove to Paris unable to make the call. Finally, he found a little café by the Eiffel Tower, pulled out his cell phone, and dialed my number.

"What?" I said.

"They terminated your deal."

I paused. "Why'd they make you fly all the way over there?"

Over the next few days, I held out hope that the Cofidis executives

would change their minds. Finally, Cofidis called and offered me about
$180,000, with a big incentive clause to pay more if I earned Inter-
national Cycling Union (ICU) bonus points based on performance in
various races. The base salary they were offering was the equivalent of
a league minimum, but it was all we had.

Bill had a Plan B. In the first week of September, there was a large
annual Interbike Expo in Anaheim, California, and all the top team
representatives would be there. Bill felt that if I showed up healthy and
announced I was ready to ride, I was sure to catch on with someone.
"Lance, we need to get in front of the press and tell everybody that
you're serious about this, and you're available," Bill said.

On September 4, 1997, I went with Bill to the Interbike Expo to
announce my return to cycling for the 1998 season. I held a press conference and drew a roomful of newspaper writers and cycling experts,
and informed them of my plans to race. I explained the Cofidis situation and made it clear that I felt jilted. I had missed a full calendar year
with cancer, and Cofidis doubted me just when I felt healthy and ready
to compete again, I said. Now the whole cycling world knew I was on
the auction block. I sat back and waited for the offers to come in.

None did.

They didn't want me. One of France's top cycling managers talked
to Bill briefly, but when he heard what Bill was asking for my services,
$500,000, he said dismissively, "That's a champion's wage. You're ex-
pecting the money of a big rider." Another team, Saeco–Cannondale,
said they might make an offer, and scheduled a meeting with Bill for
the following day. No one showed up. Bill had to go hunting for the
guy, and finally found him in another business meeting. Bill said,
"What's going on?"

The executive replied, "We can't do it."

No European team would sign me. For every twenty calls Bill put
out, maybe three were returned.

As the days went by and no one made a solid offer, I got angrier and angrier. Bill Stapleton caught the brunt of it, and it put a severe strain on our friendship. For a year and a half, he was the guy who had nothing but bad news for me. He was the person who had to tell me that I had no health insurance, that Cofidis had cut my contract. Now he had to tell me that no one wanted me.

I called my mother and told her about Cofidis, and I explained that no other team would make an offer. Not one. I could hear her tense up on the other end of the line, and the old feistiness crept into her voice.

"You know what?" she said. "That's all they've got to tell us. Because, by golly, you'll show them. They've made a terrible mistake."

All around, I encountered people who had given up on me, or who thought I was something less than I had been. One night, Kik and I went to a cocktail party with a bunch of people from the new high-tech firm she worked for. We got separated at the party, and Kik was talking across the room from me with two executives at the firm, when one of them said to her, "So that's your new boyfriend?" and then made a vulgar reference to my testicles.

"Are you sure he's good enough for you?" he said. "He's only half a man."

Kik froze. She said, "I won't even dignify that with a response, because it is so beyond not funny." She turned her back on him, and found me across the room, and told me what had happened. I was beside myself. To say something like that to her he had to be incredibly stupid, or maybe he was just a fool who drinks too much at cocktail parties, but I wasn't going to let him get away with it. I went to the bar on the pretext of getting another drink, and as I walked by him, I shouldered him, hard.

Kristin objected to my behavior, so then *we* got into an argument. I was angry way past the point of conversation. After I dropped her off at her house, I went home and sat down and composed a scathing e-mail to the guy, explaining the nature of testicular cancer and some of the statistics. I wrote dozens of different versions. "I can't believe you'd say this to anybody, let alone my girlfriend," I wrote. "And you've got a real problem if you think something like this is funny. This is a life-and-death situation. It's not about whether I have one 'nut,' or two, or fifty." But when I got done I was still upset, so I went over to Kik's house in the middle of the night, and we had a long discussion. By now she was worried that the guy would try to fire her, and we talked for a while about principles versus employment.

BILL CONTINUED TO SEARCH FOR A TEAM THAT WOULD take me on. He felt like he was running around as the agent for some B-rate swimmer that nobody wanted to talk to. People treated him like a pest. Bill just kept at it, and sheltered me from the more brutal comments. "Come on," one person said. "That guy will never ride in the peloton again. It's a joke that he could ever ride at that speed."

Finally, Bill had what he thought was a good possibility with the U.S. Postal Service team, a new organization that was American-funded and -sponsored. The chief investor in the team was Thomas Weisel, a financier from San Francisco, an old friend of mine and the former owner of the Subaru–Montgomery team. The only catch was the money. Postal, too, was offering a low base salary. Bill flew to San Francisco, and negotiations with the team's general manager, Mark Gorski, seesawed back and forth over several tense days. We were unable to reach an agreement.

I was on the verge of giving up. We still had the offer from Cofidis, but my resentment had reached the point at which I almost preferred not to race at all rather than to race for them. My disability policy was worth $20,000 a month for five years, which amounted to $1.5 million, tax-free. If I tried to race again, Lloyds of London informed Bill, I would forfeit the policy. I decided that if I was going to risk a comeback attempt, my heart should be in it. Otherwise it just didn't make sense to jeopardize my disability.

Before Bill left San Francisco, we decided he should swing by Thom Weisel's office just to say goodbye and to speak with Thom face-to-face to see if there was any chance we could work things out. Thom's office was an imposing suite in the Transamerica building with sweeping views, and Bill went there with some trepidation.

Bill sat down with Thom and Mark Gorski. Abruptly, Thom said, "Bill, what does he want?"

"He wants a base salary of $215,000," Bill said. "Also, he wants an incentive clause."

The International Cycling Union awarded bonus points on the basis of performances in big races, and if I got enough good results, I could make up in bonuses what they wouldn't pay me in salary. Bill told him I wanted $500 for every bonus point I collected up to 150, and $1,000 for every point after that.

"Would you consider a cap on the maximum number of ICU points?" Thom asked.

In a way that was a compliment, because it meant they were concerned that I might perform so well that it would cost them big money.

"No way," Bill said.

Thom stared at Bill with the long cold gaze of an expert negotiator. For weeks now, we had gotten no results at the negotiating table, and Thom Weisel was as tough and unflinching as they came. But he also knew me and believed in me. Thom opened his mouth to speak. Bill braced himself.

"I'll cover it," Thom said. "Consider it done."

Bill almost sighed aloud with relief. We had a deal; I was a racer again. I signed the agreement, and we held a big press conference to introduce me as a team member. At the press conference, I said, "I don't feel like damaged goods. I just feel out of shape, which I am." I would spend November and December training in the States, and then go overseas in January to resume racing for the first time in 18 long months. It meant returning to my old life of living out of a suitcase and riding all over the continent.

But there was a complication now: Kik. I went to Plano to see my mother. Over coffee on a Saturday morning, I said, "Let's go look at diamonds today." My mother beamed. She knew exactly what I was talking about, and we spent the day touring the best jewelers in Dallas.

I returned to Austin and planned a dinner at home for just Kik and me. We sat on the seawall behind my house, watching the sunset over Lake Austin. Finally, I said, "I have to go back to Europe, and I don't want to go without you. I want you to come with me."

The sun disappeared behind the riverbank, and dusk settled over us. It was still and dark except for the glow spilling out of my house.

I stood up. "Something came today," I said. "I want to show it to you."

I reached into my pocket and clasped the small velvet box.

"Step into the light," I said.

I opened the box, and the diamond collected the light.

"Marry me," I said.

Kik accepted.

We had never talked about my prognosis. She had come with me to my monthly checkups, and sat with me in front of those X rays, but we never felt the need to discuss the big picture. When we became engaged, however, a friend of her mother's said, "How could you let your daughter marry a cancer patient?" It forced us to think about it for the first time. Kik just said, "You know, I would rather have one year of wonderful than seventy years of mediocre. That's how I feel about it. Life's an unknown. You don't know. Nobody knows."

Kik and I packed up all our things and drove cross-country to Santa Barbara, California, where I entered an intense two-month training camp. We rented a small house on the beach, and we became so sentimental about it that we decided we wanted to be married there. We planned a wedding for May. First, however, we would move to Europe in January and spend the '98 winter and spring racing season overseas.

I got back in the gym and did basic rebuilding work, leg presses and squats, and I steadily lengthened my training rides. I surprised everyone with how well I rode during training camp in Santa Barbara. One afternoon I rode some hills with Frankie Andreu, and he said, "Man, you're killing everybody and you had cancer."

I was now officially a cancer survivor. On October 2, I had celebrated the one-year anniversary of my cancer diagnosis, which meant that I was no longer in remission. According to my doctors, there was only a minimal chance now that the disease would come back. One day, I got a note from Craig Nichols. "It's time to move on with your life," he wrote.

But how do you survive cancer? That's the part no one gives you any advice on. What does it mean? Once you finish your treatment, the doctors say, *You're cured, so go off and live. Happy trails.* But there is no support system in place to help you to deal with the emotional ramifications of trying to return to the world after being in a battle for your existence.

You don't just wake up one morning and say, "Okay, I'm done with cancer, and now it's time to go right back to the normal life I had." Stacy Pounds had proved that to me. I was physically recovered, but my soul was still healing. I was entering a phase called survivorship.

What shape was my life supposed to take? What now? What about my recurring nightmares, my dreams?

eight

SURVIVORSHIP

WHILE I WAS SICK, I TOLD MYSELF I'D NEVER cuss again, never drink another beer again, never lose my temper again. I was going to be the greatest and the most clean-living guy you could hope to meet. But life goes on. Things change, intentions get lost. You have another beer. You say another cussword.

How do you slip back into the ordinary world? That was the problem confronting me after cancer, and the old saying, that you should treat each day as if it might be your last, was no help at all. The truth is, it's a nice sentiment, but in practice it doesn't work. If I lived only for the moment, I'd be a very amiable no-account with a perpetual three-day growth on my chin. Trust me, I tried it.

People think of my comeback as a triumph, but in the beginning, it was a disaster. When you have lived for an entire year terrified of dying, you feel like you deserve to spend the rest of your days on a permanent vacation. You can't, of course; you have to return to your family, your peers, and your profession. But a part of me didn't want my old life back.

We moved to Europe in January with the U.S. Postal team. Kik quit her job, gave away her dog, leased her house, and packed up everything she owned. We rented an apartment in Cap Ferrat, halfway between Nice and Monaco, and I left her there alone while I went on the road with the team. A race wasn't an environment for wives and girlfriends. It was no different from the office; it was a job, and you didn't take your wife to the conference room.

Kristin was on her own in a foreign country, with no friends or family, and she didn't speak the language. But she reacted typically, by enrolling herself in a language-intensive French school, furnishing the apartment, and settling in as if it was a great adventure, with absolutely no sign of fear. Not once did she complain. I was proud of her.

My own attitude wasn't as good. Things weren't going so well for me on the road, where I had to adjust all over again to the hardships of racing through Europe. I had forgotten what it was like. The last time I'd been on the continent was on vacation with Kik, when we'd stayed in the best hotels and played tourists, but now it was back to the awful food, the bad beds in dingy road *pensions,* and the incessant travel. I didn't like it.

Deep down, I wasn't ready. Had I understood more about survivorship, I would have recognized that my comeback attempt was bound to be fraught with psychological problems. If I had a bad day, I had a tendency to say, "Well, I've just been through too much. I've been through three surgeries, three months of chemo, and a year of hell, and that's the reason I'm not riding well. My body is just never going to be the same." But what I really should have been saying was, "Hey, it's just a bad day."

I was riding with buried doubts, and some buried resentments, too. I was making a fraction of my old salary, and I had no new endorsements. I sarcastically called it "an eighty-percent cancer tax." I'd assumed that the minute I got back on the bike and announced a comeback, corporate America would come knocking, and when they didn't, I blamed Bill. I drove him nuts, constantly asking him why he wasn't bringing me any deals. Finally, we had a confrontation via phone—I was in Europe, he was back in Texas. I began complaining again that nothing was happening on the endorsement front.

"Look, I'll tell you what," Bill said. "I'm going to find you a new agent. I'm not putting up with this anymore. I know you think I need this, but I don't. So I quit."

I paused and said, "Well, that's not what I want."

I stopped venting on Bill, but I still brooded about the fact that no one wanted me. No European teams wanted me, and corporate America didn't want me.

My first pro race in 18 months was the Ruta del Sol, a five-day jaunt through Spain. I finished 14th, and caused a stir, but I was depressed and uncomfortable. I was used to leading, not finishing 14th. Also, I hated the attention of that first race. I felt constrained by performance anxiety and distracted by the press circus, and I wished I could have just shown up unannounced and ridden without a word, fighting through my self-doubts anonymously. I just wanted to ride in the peloton and get my legs back.

Two weeks later, I entered Paris–Nice, among the most arduous stage races outside of the Tour de France itself, an eight-day haul notorious for its wintry raw weather. Before the race itself was the "prologue," a time-trial competition. It was a seeding system of sorts; the results of the prologue would determine who rode at the front of the peloton. I finished in 19th place, not bad for a guy recovering from cancer, but I didn't see it that way. I was used to winning.

The next morning I woke up to a gray rain and blustering wind, and temperatures in the 30s. As soon as I opened my eyes I knew I didn't want to ride in that weather. I ate my breakfast morosely. I met with the team to discuss the strategy for the day, and we decided as a squad that if our team leader, George Hincapie, fell behind for any reason, we would all wait for him and help him catch up.

In the start area, I sat in a car trying to keep warm and thought about how much I didn't want to be there. When you start out thinking that way, things can't possibly get any better. Once I got out in the cold, my attitude just deteriorated. I sulked as I put on leg warmers and fought to keep some small patch of my skin dry.

We set off on a long, flat stage. The rain spit sideways, and a crosswind made it seem even colder than 35 degrees. There is nothing more demoralizing than a long flat road in the rain. At least on a climb your body stays a little bit warm because you have to work so hard, but on a flat road, you just get cold and wet to the bone. No shoe cover is good enough. No jacket is good enough. In the past, I'd thrived on being able to stand conditions that made everyone else crack. But not on this day.

Hincapie got a flat.

We all stopped. The peloton sped up the road away from us. By the time we got going again, we were 20 minutes behind the leaders, and in the wind it would take an hour of brutal effort for us to make up what we had lost. We rode off, heads down into the rain.

The crosswind cut through my clothes and made it hard to steady the bike as I churned along the side of the road. All of a sudden, I lifted my hands to the tops of the handlebars. I straightened up in my seat, and I coasted to the curb.

I pulled over. I quit. I abandoned the race. I took off my number. I thought, *This is not how I want to spend my life, freezing and soaked and in the gutter.*

Frankie Andreu was right behind me, and he remembers how I looked as I rose up and swung off the road. He could tell by the way I sat up that I might not race again for a while—if ever. Frankie told me later that his thought was "He's done."

When the rest of the team arrived back at the hotel at the end of the stage, I was packing. "I quit," I told Frankie. "I'm not racing anymore, I'm going home." I didn't care if my teammates understood or not. I said goodbye, slung my bag over my shoulder, and took off.

The decision to abandon had nothing to do with how I felt physically. I was strong. I just didn't want to be there. I simply didn't know if cycling through the cold and the pain was what I wanted to do for the rest of my life.

Kik was grocery shopping after school when I reached her on her cell phone. "I'm coming home tonight," I said. She couldn't hear because the reception wasn't great, and she said, "What? What's wrong?"

"I'll tell you about it later," I said.

"Are you hurt?" She thought I had crashed.

"No, I'm not hurt," I said. "I'll see you tonight."

A couple of hours later, Kik picked me up at the airport. We didn't say much until we got in the car and began the drive home. Finally, I said, "You know, I'm just not happy doing this."

"Why?" she said.

"I don't know how much time I have left, but I don't want to spend it cycling," I said. "I hate it. I hate the conditions. I hate being away from you. I hate this lifestyle over here. I don't want to be in Europe. I proved myself in Ruta del Sol, I showed that I could come back and do it. I have nothing left to prove to myself, or to the cancer community, so that's it."

I braced myself for her to say, "What about my school, what about my job, why did you make me move here?" But she never said it. Calmly, she said, "Well, okay."

On the plane back to Cap Ferrat I'd seen an advertisement for Harley-Davidson that summed up how I felt. It said, "If I had to live my life over again I would . . ." and then it listed several things, like, "see more sunsets." I had torn it out of the magazine, and as I explained to Kik how I felt, I handed her the ad, and I said, "This is what's wrong with cycling. It's not what my life should be."

"Well, let's get a good night's sleep, and wait a couple of days and then make a decision," she said.

The next day Kik went back to her language school, and I didn't do a thing. I sat alone in the apartment all day by myself, and I refused to even look at my bike. Kik's school had a strict rule that you weren't supposed to take phone calls. I called her three times. "I can't stand sitting around here doing nothing," I said. "I've talked to the travel agent. That's it. We're leaving."

Kik said, "I'm in class."

"I'm coming to get you. That school's a waste of time."

Kik left the classroom and sat on a bench outside, and cried. She had fought the language barrier for weeks. She had managed to set up our household, figured out how to do the marketing, and mastered the currency. She had learned how to drive the *autoroute,* and how to pay the French tolls. Now all of her effort was for nothing.

When I arrived to pick her up she was still crying. I was alarmed. "Why are you crying?" I said.

"Because we have to leave," she said.

"What do you mean? You're here with no friends. You can't speak the language. You don't have your job. Why do you want to stay here?"

"Because it's what I set out to do, and I want to finish it. But if you think we need to go home, then let's do it."

That night was a whirlwind of packing, and Kik attacked it with as much energy as she had getting us unpacked in the first place. In 24 hours we did more than most people do in two weeks. We called

Kevin Livingston, and gave him all of our stuff—towels, silverware, lamps, pots, pans, plates, vacuum cleaner. I said to Kevin, "We're never coming back. I don't want this junk." Kevin didn't try to talk me out of it—he knew better. Instead, he was very quiet. I could see on Kevin's face that he didn't think I was doing the right thing, but he wasn't going to say a word. He had always worried about my coming back, anyway. "Just watch your body," he'd say. "Take it easy." He had lived through the whole realm of the disease with me, and the only thing he cared about was my health. As I loaded him down with boxes he was so sad I thought he might cry. "Take this," I said, handing him boxes full of kitchenware. "Take all of it."

It was a nightmare, and my only good memory of that time is of Kik, and how serene she seemed in the midst of my confusion. I couldn't have blamed her if she was about to break; she had quit her job, moved to France, sacrificed everything, and almost overnight I was ready to move back to Austin and retire. But she stood by me. She was understanding and supportive and endlessly patient.

Back home in the States, everybody was wondering where I was. Carmichael was at home at eight o'clock in the morning when his phone rang. It was a French reporter. "Where is Lance Armstrong?" the reporter asked. Chris said, "He's in Paris–Nice." The reporter said in broken English, "No, he is stop." Chris hung up on him. A minute later the phone rang again—it was another French reporter.

Chris called Bill Stapleton, and Bill said he hadn't heard from me. Neither had Och. Chris tried my cell phone, and my apartment. No answer. He left messages, and I didn't return them, which was unusual.

Finally I called Chris from the airport. I said, "I'm flying home. I don't need this anymore. I don't need the crappy hotels, the weather, the lousy food. What is this doing for me?"

Chris said, "Lance, do whatever you want. But don't be rash." He continued calmly, trying to buy me a little time. "Don't talk to the press, don't announce anything, don't say you're going to quit," he warned me.

After I called Chris, I reached Stapleton. "I'm done, man," I said. "I showed them I could come back, and I'm done."

Bill kept his cool. "Okaaaay," he said. He had already talked to Chris, and he knew everything. Like Chris, he stalled.

Bill suggested that I should wait on the retirement announcement. "Let's just give it a week or so, Lance. It's too crazy right now."

"No, you don't understand. I want to do it now."

"Lance," Bill said, "I understand you're retiring. That's fine, but we need to discuss a few things. Let's just give it a couple of days."

Next, I called Och. We had one of our typical conversations.

"I quit Paris–Nice," I said.

"That's not such a big deal."

"I'm out. I'm not racing anymore."

"Don't make the decision today."

Kik and I flew back to Austin in a trail of jet lag. As we walked in the door, the phone was ringing constantly, with people looking for me and wondering why I had disappeared. Finally, things quieted down, and after a day of sleeping off the jet lag, Kik and I met with Bill in his downtown law office.

I said, "I'm not here to talk about whether I'm riding again. That's not up for discussion. I'm done, and I don't care what you think about it."

Bill looked at Kik, and she just looked back at him, and shrugged. They both knew I was in one of those moods that couldn't be argued with. By now, Kik was a shell of a woman, exhausted and frustrated, but in her glance to Bill, something passed between them. Kik's look got the point across. It said, *Be patient with him, he's a mess.*

There was about a 20-second pause before Bill spoke. Then he said, "Well, we need to at least make a statement, do this formally. Let's get it done right."

"Just issue a press release," I said. "What about that?"

"It's a bad idea."

"Why?"

"You know those races, Ruta del whatever, and Paris-whatever?" Bill said. "Nobody in America has ever heard of those, pal. Nobody here even knows you got back on a bike. So you can certainly have a press conference and tell everybody you're retired. I know you think you had this fabulous comeback, and I agree with you. I mean, what you've done is amazing. Just beating cancer is a comeback. But nobody else knows it."

"I was 14th at Ruta del Sol," I said, defensively.

"Lance," Bill said, "you will be the guy who got cancer and never rode again. That's what it's going to be."

There was another long pause. Next to me, Kik's eyes began to well up.

"Well," I said, "we can't have that."

Stapleton finessed me: he cited a thousand things that had to be done before I could formally retire. "I understand you're retiring," Bill said. "But *how* are you going to retire?" He asked me if I wanted to hold a live press conference, and suggested that we needed to have meetings with sponsors. Then he said, "Shouldn't you ride at least one farewell race?" I couldn't leave the sport without a final appearance in the U.S.

"Why not race at the national championships in June, and make that your last race?" he said. "You can win that; you know you can. *That's* a comeback; that's something people will know about."

"Well, I don't know," I said. "I don't think I want to get back on a bike."

Bill patiently manipulated me into holding off on a retirement announcement. With every complication he summoned up, he bought more time. At the very least I couldn't retire before the Ride for the Roses, he said, and that wasn't until May.

Finally, Bill wore me down. I told him I would wait to announce anything. But in the meantime, I decided I would take a few days off.

My Postal team was patient. Thom Weisel offered to wait. But a few days off turned into a week, and then a week turned into a month. I didn't even unpack my bike. It sat in its bag in the garage, collecting dust.

I WAS A BUM. I PLAYED GOLF EVERY DAY, I WATER-SKIED, I drank beer, and I lay on the sofa and channel-surfed.

I went to Chuy's for Tex-Mex, and violated every rule of my training diet. Whenever I came home from Europe, it was a tradition for me to stop at Chuy's straight from the airport, no matter how jet-lagged I was, and order a burrito with tomatillo sauce and a couple of margaritas or Shiner Bocks. Now I was eating practically every meal there. I never intended to deprive myself again; I'd been given a second chance and I was determined to take advantage of it.

But it wasn't fun. It wasn't lighthearted or free or happy. It was forced. I tried to re-create the mood I'd shared with Kik on our European vacation, but this time, things were different, and I couldn't understand why. The truth was, I felt ashamed. I was filled with self-doubt and embarrassed by what I'd done in Paris–Nice. *Son, you never quit.* But I'd quit.

I was behaving totally out of character, and the reason was survivorship. It was a classic case of "Now what?" I'd had a job and a life, and then I got sick, and it turned my life upside-down, and when I

tried to go back to my life I was disoriented, nothing was the same—
and I couldn't handle it.

I hated the bike, but I thought, *What else am I going to do? Be a coffee boy in an office?* I didn't exactly feel like a champ at much else. I
didn't know what to do, so for the moment, I just wanted to escape,
and that's what I did. I evaded my responsibilities.

I know now that surviving cancer involved more than just a con-
valescence of the body. My mind and my soul had to convalesce,
too.

No one quite understood that—except for Kik. She kept her composure when she had every right to be distraught and furious with me
for pulling the rug out from under her. While I was out playing golf
every day, she was homeless, dogless, and jobless, reading the classifieds
and wondering how we were going to support ourselves. My mother
sympathized with what she was going through. She would call us, ask
to speak with Kik, and say, "How are *you* doing?"

But after several weeks of the golf, the drinking, the Mexican food,
Kik decided it was enough—somebody had to try to get through to
me. One morning we were sitting outside on the patio having coffee.
I put down my cup and said, "Well, okay, I'll see you later. It's my tee
time."

"Lance," Kik said, "what am *I* doing today?"

"What do you mean?"

"You didn't ask me what I was going to do today. You didn't ask me
what I wanted to do, or if I minded if you played golf. You just told
me what you were going to do. Do you care what I'm doing?"

"Oh, sorry," I said.

"What am I doing today?" she said. "What am I doing? Tell me
that."

I was silent. I didn't know what to say.

"You need to decide something," she told me. "You need to decide if you are going to retire for real, and be a golf-playing, beer-drinking, Mexican-food-eating slob. If you are, that's fine. I love you, and I'll marry you anyway. But I just need to know, so I can get myself together and go back on the street, and get a job to support your golfing. Just tell me.

"But if you're not going to retire, then you need to stop eating and drinking like this and being a bum, and you need to figure it out, because you are deciding by not deciding, and that is so un–Lance. It is just not you. And I'm not quite sure who you are right now. I love you anyway, but you need to figure something out."

She wasn't angry as she said it. She was just right: I didn't really know what I was trying to accomplish, and I was just being a bum. All of a sudden I saw a reflection of myself as a retiree in her eyes, and I didn't like it. She wasn't going to live an idle life, and I didn't blame her.

Quietly, she said, "So tell me if we're going to stay in Austin. If so, I'm going to get a job, because I'm not going to sit at home while you play golf. I'm so bored."

Normally, nobody could talk to me like that. But she said it almost sweetly, without fighting. Kik knew how stubborn I could be when someone tried to butt heads with me; it was my old reflex against control and authority. I don't like to be cornered, and when I am, I will fight my way out, whether physically or logically or emotionally. But as she spoke to me I didn't feel attacked or defensive, or hurt, or picked on, I just knew the honest truth when I heard it. It was, in a quietly sarcastic way, a very profound conversation. I stood up from the table.

"Okay," I said. "Let me think about it."

I went to play golf anyway, because I knew Kik didn't mind that. Golf wasn't the issue. The issue was finding myself again.

Kik and Stapleton and Carmichael and Och conspired against me, talking constantly behind my back about how to get me back on the bike. I continued to say that I was retiring, but as the days wore on, I began to waver. Bill persuaded me to commit to one last race, the U.S. Pro Championships, which would be held in Philadelphia in May.

Chris Carmichael flew to Austin. He took one look in my garage, at the bike still in its carrying bag, and shook his head. Chris felt like Kik did, that I needed to make a conscious decision about whether I belonged back on the bike. "You're alive again, and now you need to get back to living," he repeated. But he knew I wasn't ready to commit to another full-scale comeback yet, so the surface excuse he gave for coming to Austin was simply to put together a training plan for the U.S. Championships. Also, the second Ride for the Roses was coming up, and the race would be a criterium around downtown Austin requiring that I be at least minimally fit. "You can't go out like this," Chris said, gesturing at my body. "You don't want to embarrass your foundation."

Chris insisted that regardless of what I decided about retirement, I needed an eight- to ten-day intensive training camp to get back to form—and I needed to do it somewhere other than Austin. "Let's get out of town," he said. "You can't focus here, there's too much golf, too many distractions."

We tried to think of a place to go. Arizona? Too hot. Colorado? Too high altitude. Then I said, "Remember Boone? That little hippie town in North Carolina?"

Boone was high in the Appalachians on the route of the old Tour Du Pont, and I had fond memories of it. I had won the Tour Du Pont twice there, and I had spent many afternoons cycling and suffering on its biggest peak, Beech Mountain, which was the crucial climbing stage of the race. It was arduous but beautiful country, and Boone itself was a college town full of students and professors from nearby Appalachian State University. Conveniently, it had a training facility at the university, and plenty of cabins for rent in the woods.

I got on the Internet and rented a cabin sight unseen. Next, I decided to invite an old friend named Bob Roll to be my training partner; Bob was a high-spirited 38-year-old former road racer who had switched over to mountain biking, and he would be easy company for ten days.

We flew to Charlotte, North Carolina, and drove three hours into the mountains. Our first stop was Appalachian State, where Chris arranged with the athletic training center to do some testing with me on a stationary bike, to find out where I stood fitness-wise. Chris looked at my VO_2 max and lactate threshold numbers, and they confirmed what he already knew: I was fat and in lousy shape. Usually, my physiological values were the elite of the elite. My VO_2 rate, ordinarily at 85, was now at 64.

Chris said to the Appalachian State trainers who helped us, "Watch. When we come back he's going to be at 74, and he'll do it after only a week."

Chris knew that my body responded to new thresholds after a very short period, and he felt I could be back in peak shape in just a few days. But just to challenge me, he made me a bet that I couldn't up my wattage—the amount of work in pedaling—in the space of a week. "A hundred bucks says you can't get over 500," he said. I took the bet.

From then on, all we did was eat, sleep, and ride bikes. Spring had just begun moving up into the mountains, creating a constant fog and drizzle that seemed to muffle the piney woods. We rode in the rain every day. The cold seared my lungs, and with every breath I blew out a stream of white frost, but I didn't mind. It made me feel clean. We rode winding back roads, only some of which were paved and mapped. We cycled over gravel and hardpan and beds of pine needles, and under hanging boughs.

At night, Chris made big pots of pasta and baked potatoes and we sat around the table wolfing down the food and having unprintable conversations. We told stories and laughed about old times and the start of our friendship, and my first years as a pro.

I called home each night, and Kristin could tell that I was starting to sound like my old self; I was having fun, joking, I didn't seem depressed. When I would tell her about the cold and rainy weather or how far we had ridden, I would laugh. "I'm feeling really good," I said, almost puzzled.

I began to enjoy the single-mindedness of training, riding hard during the day and holing up in the cabin in the evenings. I even appreciated the awful weather. It was as if I was going back to Paris–Nice and staring the elements that had defeated me in the eye. What had cracked me in Paris were the cold, wet conditions, but now I took satisfaction in riding through them, the way I'd used to.

Toward the end of the camp, we decided to ride Beech Mountain. Chris knew exactly what he was doing when he suggested it, because there was a time when I owned that mountain. It was a strenuous 5,000-foot climb with a snowcapped summit, and it had been the crucial stage in my two Tour Du Pont victories. I remembered laboring on up the mountainside with crowds lined along the route, and how they had painted my name across the road: "Go Armstrong."

We set out on yet another cold, raining, foggy day with a plan to ride a 100-mile loop before we returned and undertook the big finishing ascent of Beech Mountain. Chris would follow in a car, so we could load the bikes up on the rack after we reached the summit and drive back to the cabin for dinner.

We rode and rode through a steady rain, for four hours, and then five. By the time we got to the foot of Beech, I'd been on the bike for six hours, drenched. But I lifted myself up out of the saddle and propelled the bike up the incline, leaving Bob Roll behind.

As I started up the rise, I saw an eerie sight: the road still had my name painted on it.

My wheels spun over the washed-out old yellow and white lettering. I glanced down between my feet. It said, faintly, *Viva Lance.*

I continued upward, and the mountain grew steeper. I hammered down on the pedals, working hard, and felt a small bloom of sweat and satisfaction, a heat under my skin almost like a liquor blush. My body reacted instinctively to the climb. Mindlessly, I rose out of my seat and picked up the pace. Suddenly, Chris pulled up behind me in the follow car, rolled down his window, and began driving me on. "Go, go, go!" he yelled. I glanced back at him. *"Allez Lance, allez, allez!"* he yelled. I mashed down on the pedals, heard my breath grow shorter, and I accelerated.

That ascent triggered something in me. As I rode upward, I reflected on my life, back to all points, my childhood, my early races, my illness, and how it changed me. Maybe it was the primitive act of climbing that made me confront the issues I'd been evading for weeks. It was time to quit stalling, I realized. *Move,* I told myself. *If you can still move, you aren't sick.*

I looked again at the ground as it passed under my wheels, at the water spitting off the tires and the spokes turning round. I saw more faded painted letters, and I saw my washed-out name: *Go Armstrong.*

As I continued upward, I saw my life as a whole. I saw the pattern and the privilege of it, and the purpose of it, too. It was simply this: I was meant for a long, hard climb.

I approached the summit. Behind me, Chris could see in the attitude of my body on the bike that I was having a change of heart. Some weight, he sensed, was simply no longer there.

Lightly, I reached the top of the mountain. I cruised to a halt. Chris put the car in park and got out. We didn't talk about what had just happened. Chris just looked at me, and said, "I'll put your bike on top of the car."

"No," I said. "Give me my rain jacket. I'm riding back."

I was restored. I was a bike racer again. Chris smiled and got back in the car.

I passed the rest of the trip in a state of near-reverence for those beautiful, peaceful, soulful mountains. The rides were demanding and quiet, and I rode with a pure love of the bike, until Boone began to feel like the Holy Land to me, a place I had come to on a pilgrimage. If I ever have any serious problems again, I know that I will go back to Boone and find an answer. I got my life back on those rides.

A day or two later we went to the university training center to test my wattage. I pedaled so hard I blew out the odometer. I spun the machine so fast Chris couldn't get a digital readout. Laughing, he smacked $100 into my palm.

That night at dinner, I said to Chris casually, "I wonder if I could get into that race in Atlanta."

"Let's do it," Chris said.

That evening, we started figuring out my comeback. Chris placed a bunch of calls, trying to find me some new racing wheels. Then he called Bill Stapleton, and said, "Get ready. He's coming back a different guy. The guy we used to know."

I DIDN'T JUST JUMP BACK ON THE BIKE AND WIN. THERE were a lot of ups and downs, good results and bad results, but this time I didn't let the lows get to me.

After Boone, I enjoyed every day on the bike. Every day. Even when I was in bad shape, suffering, crashing, trying to come back, I never once, never, ever, ever, thought about abandoning again.

I even took the bike to my wedding. My trip to Boone was in April of '98, and Kik and I were married that May in Santa Barbara. We invited about a hundred people, and we exchanged vows in a small Catholic ceremony—Kik is Catholic—and afterward we had a dance party. No one sat down for the duration of the night, people were too busy rocking all over the room, and it was such a good time that Kik and I didn't want it to end. We ended up in the hotel bar with our guests in our wedding getups, and had cocktails and cigars.

We stayed on in a beach house for a few days, but it wasn't the ideal honeymoon, because I was so intent on training after my Boone experience. I rode every day. Finally we returned home to Austin for the Ride for the Roses, which had grown to be a big-time event. Part of downtown was blocked off, lights were strung up through the streets. I won the criterium over a pretty good field. When I took the podium, Kik shrieked and jumped around, as thrilled as if it were the Tour de France. It struck me that she had never seen me win anything before. "That's nothing," I said, shrugging, but I was secretly delighted.

It was nice to have a little taste of competition again. I got another in June, when I made my official return to the cycling circuit and finished fourth in the U.S. Pro Championships, while my friend and teammate George Hincapie won it.

One morning I said to Kik, "Okay, maybe it's time to try Europe again." She just nodded cheerfully and started packing. The thing is, I could have said to her: "We're going back to Europe," and when we got to Europe, I could have said, "We're going back to Austin," and when we got to Austin, I could have said, "You know what? I made a mistake. We're going back to Europe," and she would have made every trip without complaint. Nothing was a huge crisis to her.

Kik liked the challenge of a new place and a new language, so

when I said: "Okay, let's try it one more time," that was an easy one for
her. Some wives would have thought it was hard, but that's why I
didn't marry some wives. A lot of wives wouldn't have made it over
there in the first place. My wife, on the other hand, is a stud.

Kik and I tentatively rented a little apartment in Nice, and she en-
rolled back in school and started French lessons again, while I continued to race. I entered the Tour of Luxembourg—and I won it. After
the first stage, I called home, and Kik wanted to know why I wasn't
more excited, but by now I was so wary of the psychological pitfalls
of a comeback that I kept my emotions and expectations in check. It
was just a four-day race, not the kind that the major riders would have
celebrated as a big victory. But from a morale standpoint it was great,
because it meant I could win again—and it was worth some ICU
bonus points, too. It erased the last lingering bit of self-doubt.

Next, I traveled to the weeklong Tour of Holland, and finished
fourth. In July, I skipped the Tour de France, not yet ready for the
strenuous routine of a three-week stage race. Instead, I did some TV
commentary and watched from the side of the road as it turned into
the most controversial and traumatic bike race in history. In a series of
raids on team cars, French police found trunkloads of EPO and ana-
bolic steroids. Team members and officials were thrown in French
jails, everyone was under suspicion, and the cyclists were furious at the
tactics used by authorities. Of the 21 teams that began the race, only
14 finished. One team was expelled and the other six quit in protest.

Doping is an unfortunate fact of life in cycling, or any other endurance sport for that matter. Inevitably, some teams and riders feel it's
like nuclear weapons—that they have to do it to stay competitive
within the peloton. I never felt that way, and certainly after chemo the
idea of putting anything foreign in my body was especially repulsive.
Overall, I had extremely mixed feelings about the 1998 Tour: I sympathized with the riders caught in the firestorm, some of whom I

knew well, but I also felt the Tour would be a more fair event from then on.

I continued to make steady progress on the bike through the summer, and in August Kik and I felt secure enough about my future as a rider to buy a house in Nice. While Kik employed her stumbling French to handle the bankers and buy furniture and move us into the new home, I went off with the team for the three-week Vuelta a España (Tour of Spain), one of the most strenuous races on the face of the earth. There are three grand tours in cycling, of Italy, Spain, and France.

On October 1, 1998, nearly two years to the day after I was diagnosed, I completed the Vuelta. I finished fourth, and it was as important an achievement as any race I'd ever won. I rode 2,348 miles over 23 days, and missed making the awards podium by only six seconds. The winner, Abraham Olano of Spain, had ridden just 2 minutes and 18 seconds faster than I had. What's more, I nearly won the toughest mountain stage of the race, in gale-force winds and freezing temperatures. The race was so tough that almost half the field retired before the finish. But I didn't quit.

To place fourth in the Vuelta meant more than just a comeback. In my previous life, I'd been a great one-day racer, but I'd never been competitive in a three-week stage race. The Vuelta meant I was not only back, I was *better.* I was capable of winning any race in the world. I swept up ICU ranking points right and left, and all of a sudden I was the real deal.

WHILE I WAS RIDING IN THE VUELTA, KIK WAS IN AN endurance contest of her own called moving. Our apartment was on the third floor, and she would call up the elevator, load it with our things—boxes of clothes, cycling gear, and kitchenware. She would ride down and unload everything in the lobby, and then she'd move it all from the lobby to the front door of the building, and from there into the back of the car. She'd drive to the new house, unload the car, carry the boxes up a set of steep stairs ascending a hillside, and dump them in the house. Then she'd drive back to the apartment and repeat the routine all over again, elevator load by elevator load. Kik worked for two days straight, until she was bleary-eyed with fatigue.

When I arrived home, my clothes were put away, the refrigerator was full of groceries, and Kik handed me a new set of keys. For some reason, it made me ridiculously happy. That house seemed like the culmination of the whole year. We had done it, we had established ourselves in Europe and regained my career. Kik could speak some French now, and we had a home and a life together, and it meant everything to us. "Oh, my God," she said. "We did it. We started over."

To celebrate we spent a few days in Lake Como, which was still one of my favorite places anywhere. I treated us to a wonderful hotel, and handpicked the room we stayed in, with a gigantic terrace and sweeping view, and all we did was sleep and stroll and go to elegant dinners.

Finally, we went home to Austin for the fall and winter holidays. Not long after we got back, I received an e-mail from the U.S. Postal team director, Johan Bruyneel. He congratulated me on the Vuelta. "I think that fourth was better than you expected," he wrote. Then he made an interesting reference. "You will look great on the podium of the Tour de France next year," Johan wrote, cryptically.

That was the end of the message. I saved his e-mail to a disk, printed it out, and looked at the words. The Tour? Johan didn't just think I could be a stage racer again, he thought I could be a Tour rider. He thought I could win the whole thing.

It was worth considering.

Over the next few days, I read and reread the e-mail. After a year of confusion and self-doubt, I now knew exactly what I should do.

I wanted to win the Tour de France.

WHAT YOU LEARN IN SURVIVORSHIP IS THAT AFTER ALL the shouting is done, after the desperation and crisis is over, after you have accepted the fact of your illness and celebrated the return of your health, the old routines and habits, like shaving in the morning with a purpose, a job to go to, and a wife to love and a child to raise, these are the threads that tie your days together and that give them the pattern deserving of the term "a life."

One of the things I loved about Boone was the view it offered. When I cycled around an unexpected bend in the road, suddenly the landscape opened up, the line of trees parted, and I could see thirty mountain ranges stretching to the horizon. I was beginning to see my life in the same way.

I wanted to have a child. When I was sick, fatherhood was something obscured around the next bend, perhaps impossible, a lost chance. Now my view was as clear and crystallized as those mountain ranges in the distance, and I didn't want to postpone fatherhood any longer. Fortunately, Kik was as ready as I was. We understood each other perfectly despite the upheavals of the last year, and we'd held on to a sweet harmony, the kind that makes you want to join with another and create a new human being.

Ironically, the process would be almost as medically intricate as a cancer treatment: it would require as much research and planning, and a raft of syringes, drugs, and two surgeries. I was sterile. In order to get pregnant, Kik would need in-vitro fertilization (IVF), using the sperm I had banked in San Antonio on that awful day.

What follows in these pages is an attempt to render the experience truthfully and openly. A lot of couples are private about their IVF treatment and don't want to talk about it at all, which is their right. We aren't. We understand we may be criticized for being so free with the details, but we have decided to share them because so many couples deal with infertility and are faced with the fear that they may not be able to have a family. We want them to hear the specifics of IVF so they understand what's ahead of them. For us, it was forbidding but worth it.

We planned to start our family right after the New Year, and I began to research in-vitro as thoroughly as cancer, scouring the Internet and consulting with physicians. We scheduled a trip to New York City to visit the IVF experts at Cornell University. But as the date drew closer on the calendar, we started having second thoughts. The experience was going to be clinical and impersonal enough, and we were so tired of travel that the idea of being in a strange hotel room for weeks in New York sounded as unappealing as a chemo cycle. We changed course and decided to seek an IVF specialist at home in Austin, Dr. Thomas Vaughn.

On December 28, we had our first consultation with Dr. Vaughn. Both of us were nervous as we sat on the couch in his office, and out of habit I wore what Kik called my "medical demeanor," which I put on in any clinical situation, a tight-lipped, hard look. Kik smiled a lot to offset my grimness, so Dr. Vaughn would think we were fit to be parents.

As we discussed the IVF procedure, I noticed Kik blushed slightly. She wasn't used to the clinical language, but after testicular cancer, discussing sexual matters publicly with strangers was no big deal to me. We left the office with a rough plan in place and a sense of surprise that it could happen so fast—if things worked, Kik could be pregnant by February. The timing was important, because we'd have to plan the arrival of the new baby along with my cycling schedule if I wanted to win the Tour de France.

Two days later, Kik went to an X-ray lab for her first appointment. Nurses strapped her to a sliding X-ray table and stuck a torture device inside her that sprayed dye. The X ray was to make sure she didn't have any blocked tubes or other problems. Well, the nurses messed up twice before they finally got it right, and it hurt Kik to the point that she sobbed. But, typical Kik, she was impatient with herself for crying. "I'm so pathetic," she said.

The next night was New Year's Eve, the last night of libations for her. As of the New Year she forswore alcohol and caffeine. The following morning my Java Queen nursed a hangover and caffeine withdrawal, and from then on she didn't touch a drop. We wanted our baby to be pristine.

A week later, we had an appointment at the hospital for what we thought was a simple meeting with an IVF nurse. Wrong. We walked into the room and it was, no joke, staged like an intervention. Two long tables faced each other, with tense couples holding hands in utter silence. A too-chipper nurse said she had to take our photo for her files, so we gritted our teeth and smiled, and we sat down for two hours of Sex Ed, complete with old films of sperm swimming up the tubes. We'd all seen it in high school, and we didn't want to see it again. The nurses handed out information packets and proceeded to go through them page by page. I squirmed in my seat, and kept Kik amused by drawing pictures of a sperm with a circle and a slash through it, and whispering jokes. I told Kik I felt like I was at an Al-Anon meeting: "Hi, my name is Lance and I have no sperm."

I elbowed Kik to go, but there was never a good time to leave. We both sat there, dying to bolt, but we couldn't find the right, polite break. Finally we couldn't take one more minute. Kik gathered her pamphlets, stood up, and race-walked out of the room with me right on her wheel. We burst out of the room, giddy as school kids, and ran to our car laughing and out of breath, and wondered aloud if we were too immature to be parents.

A few days later we returned to the IVF office for blood tests. Kik turned bedsheet white when she had her blood drawn. I told her she was a skirt, but I actually sympathized. She has needle-phobia—and she was in for a rough few weeks.

That night she took her first Lupron shot. Lupron is a drug that prevents women from ovulating, and she required ten units every 24 hours—which meant a shot every night until the doctors told her to stop. For someone with an aversion to needles, those shots were highly unnerving. To make matters worse, she had to administer them to herself.

Every night at exactly 8:30 P.M., Kik had to go into the bathroom and give herself a shot in the thigh. The first time she did it, her hands shook so badly that she couldn't get the tiny bubbles out of the syringe. Finally she pinched her thigh hard, swore out loud, and stuck herself.

In the middle of the week, the U.S. Postal team came to Austin to do wind-tunnel testing. Kik and I took everybody out to dinner, but just as the entrées arrived Kik looked at her watch. It was 8:30 P.M. She excused herself, and went to the bathroom and "shot up like some junkie," as she delicately put it.

After wind-tunnel testing, the U.S. Postal team went to California for a training camp and I had to go with them, which meant Kik would be alone in the pregnancy project for several days. While I was away, Kik made a grand pilgrimage to the clinic in San Antonio where my frozen sperm was stored. I had been paying rent on it, $100 every year.

Early that morning, Kik went to the IVF office in Austin and picked up a big frozen tank, which filled the passenger seat next to her. She drove an hour to San Antonio and lugged the tank inside the building and up to the 13th floor, where she read a *House Beautiful* magazine while one of the nurses prepared our family for the icy trip back to Austin. At my request, the nurse opened the tank briefly to show Kik the initials *LA* etched into the vial.

"I said a silent prayer that the vial didn't belong to some guy named Larry Anderson," she told me later.

On her way back she drove very carefully and answered several inquiring calls from me, checking her progress. I didn't feel quite safe until she had deposited the tank back into the hands of the IVF staff. It was not quite the romantic candlelight interlude we had in mind, but we were now prepared to conceive a child.

Kik continued to shoot herself up. One night she had a bunch of girlfriends to the house for dinner, and when 8:30 came around none of them could believe she was actually going to stick herself with a needle, so they joined her in the master bath to watch. Call it stage fright, call it slippery fingers—but she dropped her last glass vial of Lupron on the bathroom tile and it shattered. She stared at it, disbelieving and horrified, knowing full well that if she missed her shot, she would also miss the entire cycle and have to start all over again in another month. Her eyes filled up with tears. While her friends cleaned up the shards before the dog ate them, Kik frantically searched through her info binder for the name of the nurse on call, and reached her. It was 8:45 on a Saturday night, and Kik tearfully explained the situation. The nurse said, "Oh, dear." They both called around town to find a pharmacy that was open. Finally Kik found one, and raced down the freeway. The pharmacist kept the store open, waited for her to arrive, and gave her a good-luck pat as she left.

A couple of days later, Kik went back to Dr. Vaughn for a baseline sonogram to count and measure her eggs. It was hard for Kik to go to the doctor by herself. All of the other women at the clinic always had their husbands with them, and she could feel them looking at her as she leafed through *People* magazine. She read their thoughts: they wondered why someone so young would need IVF, and why she was always alone.

Doctor Vaughn started her on Gonal-F. This was the drug that would stimulate the follicle and make her produce more eggs. From now on she would have to take *two* shots: five units of Lupron and three full vials of Gonal-F. She told me that her body, once a temple, was now "a cross between a pincushion and a henhouse."

Mixing the Gonal-F was hard to do. It came in powder form in glass vials. Kik had to take a syringe with a long needle, which made her ill just to look at, and draw a half-unit of a sterile water solution. Then she broke the tops off the vials of powder and shot the liquid into each vial. She filled the syringe with the mixture, flicked it to remove a fat air bubble at the top, and squirted until the air pocket moved up and out of the needle. Then she injected the evil needle's contents into her thigh.

On January 22, Kik went to Dr. Vaughn at 7 A.M. to have blood drawn yet again. Another needle. She looked as far away from it as possible and focused on the Far Side cartoons taped to the wall, wondering how she was going to handle childbirth if she couldn't even give blood without feeling woozy. Then, at 4 P.M. the same day, she went *back* to Dr. Vaughn's office to get her second sonogram. It revealed 12 eggs, all of them growing right on schedule.

It was the height of irony: on the same day that she had the sonogram, I went from California to Oregon to see Dr. Nichols for my six-month cancer checkup. Dr. Nichols had moved from Indianapolis to Portland, but I continued to visit him for my periodic monitoring. I couldn't help remarking on the fact that while I was seeing one kind of doctor, she was seeing another, for entirely different purposes. But we told ourselves they had one thing in common: each confirmed the possibility of life.

Kik was almost ready for "retrieval," the surgery to harvest her eggs. The day before she was due to have the procedure I arrived back home, to our mutual relief. That day she underwent one more round of blood tests and sonograms, and yet another shot, a dose of HCG, the blood marker that had haunted my life during chemo. In this case, HCG was a good thing; it would mature the egg in Kik's body for retrieval.

She had the shot at exactly 7:30 P.M., 36 hours before surgery, at a local clinic. It was the longest needle yet, but a very gentle nurse administered the shot while Kik lay on a table quivering.

That night, she dreamed of knives and henhouses.

On the day of the procedure, we rose at 6 A.M. and went to the day-surgery center, where Kik was given hospital attire to change into, complete with a blue shower cap and patient's gown. The anesthesiologist explained his procedure and handed us a stack of releases to sign. Nervously, we scribbled our names on each of them, including one that gave the doctors the right to cut open her abdomen to retrieve the eggs if the traditional way of extracting them via a needle didn't work. Then Kik walked into the surgery room.

She was literally strapped to a table, with her arms outstretched like a crucifixion. She doesn't remember anything after the anesthesia IV began. It's a good thing. The doctor harvested her eggs using a very long needle and a catheter.

When she woke up in the recovery room, she saw me leaning over her. "Will you get in bed with me?" she asked. I crawled in next to her, and kept her company while she dozed on and off for another hour. Finally she woke up, and the hospital released us. I pushed her in a wheelchair out to our car, and for only the second time in my life, I drove the speed limit home.

Kik spent the weekend resting, sleeping, and watching movies while I cooked and looked after her. Bart Knaggs' wife, Barbara, came by with some flowers and handed us a carton of eggs. "Since you no longer have any," she said. It hurt Kik to laugh, but it didn't hurt as badly as the progesterone shot I gave her. The latest doctor's order was a nightly dose of progesterone, and this was the longest and most oily-looking needle yet. I had to do it for her.

On February 1, Dr. Vaughn called with our fertilization report. They had defrosted the frozen sperm and fertilized Kik's eggs via a procedure called intracytoplasmic sperm injection (ICSI), whereby they physically injected one sperm into each egg. We had nine viable eggs, he said. Of those nine, six were perfect, two were possible, and one was broken. We decided to implant three of the perfect ones in Kik's womb, and to freeze the other three. It was strange to think that we were freezing our future children.

After we hung up, we had a moment of panic. I wondered aloud, "What would we would do if all three *worked?*" We could end up with three screaming, scampering, spoon-banging toddlers all at the same time.

Three days after the retrieval, we went back to the hospital for the "transfer," which was the clinical, bus-station term for what we considered the most important day in our lives apart from our wedding. We were ushered to the day-surgery area, where our embryologist, Beth Williamson, explained that she had spent the weekend fertilizing our embryos. She said that when she thawed the sperm she was happy to find that they were alive and swimming, which was a relief because this is not always the case after cryo-preservation. She said the fertilization went smoothly—and she even had photos for us. "Here's the group shot," she said, which was her hilarious term for a fuzzy image of three embryos together, followed by individual shots of each. The embryos had eight cells, and they were dividing right on schedule.

"Can you tell the gender?" Kik asked.

Dr. Williamson said no, that the gender at this stage could only be determined by removing one of the cells and doing DNA testing. I'd had enough procedures to last me a lifetime. "Uh, no thanks," I said. "We'd rather be curious."

After Beth left, a nurse came in with two sets of scrubs—one for Kik and one for me. As we got dressed, Kik said, "You look like some hunk from *ER."* Giggling, we asked Dr. Vaughn to take a picture of us, to mark our last moment as a couple without children. Then we went into a darkened surgery room. The lights were dimmed to make everything as relaxing as possible. We weren't anxious; we were only very excited, and both grinning like idiots. Finally, the doctor indicated to the embryologist team that it was time, and they came in with our three embryos in a syringe. I sat on a stool next to Kik, and I held both of her hands under the sheet. Within five minutes it was complete. We never took our eyes off of each other.

Next, the team lifted Kik very carefully onto a gurney and wheeled her into the small recovery room, where she had to lie motionless for one hour. I sprawled out on a bed next to her. We just lay there together, looking up at the ceiling, and teasing each other about having triplets.

After our hour was up, a nurse came in and explained that Kik would have to spend the next two days doing absolutely nothing. I drove carefully home, and put her in bed, and waited on her. I delivered her lunch on a tray, and for dinner I set the table with pretty cloth napkins.

"Armstrong, party of five," I announced.

I served dinner like a headwaiter. Kik was only allowed to sit up while we ate, and in between the salad and the main course I made her lie down on the sofa. She dubbed me "the warden."

Kik woke up the next morning to me kissing her stomach. That day she began taking medications we called "hatching drugs." The embryology team had poked a microscopic hole in each of the fertilized follicles before they transferred them, and the hatching drugs, along with that tiny hole, would help the embryos hatch out of the follicle and implant.

We wouldn't know for two weeks, until February 15, whether Kik was actually pregnant, and we could barely wait. We kept trying to notice any subtle changes in the way she felt. But considering that she had been taking shots and pills for weeks on end, it was hard to make a comparison to "normal." "Do you feel anything different?" I kept asking, anxiously. "What is it supposed to feel like?" We wondered about it all the time.

"Am I?" she'd say.

Finally, on the eleventh day after the transplant, Kik went back to the hospital early in the morning to have blood drawn for her HCG (pregnancy) test. She was so nervous that she turned the radio off and prayed to herself on the way there and back. The results would be back by 1:30 P.M., so we tried to pass the time by fixing a big breakfast, showering, and packing for Europe.

Just as Kik was taking the dog out for a walk, the phone rang. I picked it up and I said, "Uh-huh," and listened, and my eyes filled with tears. I hung up the phone, and I grabbed her in a huge hug, and I said, "Babe, you're pregnant." Kik threw her arms around me and said, "Are you *sure?*" I laughed, and then we both cried.

Now that we knew she was pregnant, the question became, how many babies was she carrying? I cheerfully announced that I hoped she was carrying triplet boys. "The more the better," I said.

Kik rolled her eyes. "My husband has a rich fantasy life," she said. "Either that or he finds humor in tormenting me."

"I picture you on an eleven-hour international flight with the triplets," I said. "See also: insanity, fatigue, catatonic state, insomnia."

Kik was sure to do everything carefully. She ate from all the major food groups, she walked four miles a day, she took her prenatal vitamins, and she napped. She bought a stack of pregnancy books, and we looked at cribs. Friends kept asking if she had been sick yet, which she hadn't. In fact, she felt so good that she began to wonder if maybe the hospital mixed up her blood test and she wasn't pregnant after all.

She did a home pregnancy test just to ease her fears. Two lines popped right up.

"Okay, just checking," she said.

Finally, I had to return to Europe and the U.S. Postal team. Kik stayed behind for a couple more tests, but she would join me overseas as soon as possible. On March 5, she had a sonogram to judge the number of babies she was carrying. I had almost convinced her that she was going to bear triplet boys—but the sonogram showed that we had one healthy baby. Not twins, not triplets. She was relieved, but a tiny part of her was oddly disappointed, not because she wanted us to be the parents of multiples, but because she couldn't ignore the vague loss she felt, wondering what happened to the other two. Kik asked Dr. Vaughn if there was any possible thing we could have done wrong that might have kept the other two from living. He said absolutely not, and that there are still some things that are natural and inexplicable, even in a seemingly sterile, scientific procedure.

Then Dr. Vaughn said, "That's quite a strong heartbeat we have here."

He pointed to a tiny blinking bean on the screen. The entire thing was flashing. Kik laughed and said, "It definitely isn't my genes that made a heart beat like that. That's Lance." Dr. Vaughn printed out an obscure photo of the bean for Kik to take to Europe for me.

A couple of days later, Kik arrived in Nice. She handed me the picture. I studied it, awestruck, absolutely mesmerized. That bean with a flashing heartbeat made me feel more alive than anything I had experienced yet. It made me feel as clean and reverent as Boone. It made me feel as if I had survived, at last.

"Ride like the wind," Kik told me. "Big Daddy Armstrong has a family to support."

nine

THE TOUR

LIFE IS LONG—HOPEFULLY. BUT "LONG" IS A
relative term: a minute can seem like a month when you're pedaling
uphill, which is why there are few things that seem longer than the
Tour de France. How long is it? Long as a freeway guardrail stretching into shimmering, flat-topped oblivion. Long as fields of parched
summer hay with no fences in sight. Long as the view of three nations
from atop an icy, jagged peak in the Pyrenees.

It would be easy to see the Tour de France as a monumentally inconsequential undertaking: 200 riders cycling the entire circumference
of France, mountains included, over three weeks in the heat of the
summer. There is no reason to attempt such a feat of idiocy, other than
the fact that some people, which is to say some people like me, have

a need to search the depths of their stamina for self-definition. (I'm the guy who can take it.) It's a contest in purposeless suffering.

But for reasons of my own, I think it may be the most gallant athletic endeavor in the world. To me, of course, it's about living.

A little history: the bicycle was an invention of the industrial revolution, along with the steam engine and the telegraph, and the first Tour was held in 1903, the result of a challenge in the French sporting press issued by the newspaper *L'Auto*. Of the sixty racers who started, only 21 finished, and the event immediately captivated the nation. An estimated 100,000 spectators lined the roads into Paris, and there was cheating right from the start: drinks were spiked, and tacks and broken bottles were thrown onto the road by the leaders to sabotage the riders chasing them. The early riders had to carry their own food and equipment, their bikes had just two gears, and they used their feet as brakes. The first mountain stages were introduced in 1910 (along with brakes), when the peloton rode through the Alps, despite the threat of attacks from wild animals. In 1914, the race began on the same day that the Archduke Ferdinand was shot. Five days after the finish of the race, war swept into the same Alps the riders had climbed.

Today, the race is a marvel of technology. The bikes are so light you can lift them overhead with one hand, and the riders are equipped with computers, heart monitors, and even two-way radios. But the essential test of the race has not changed: who can best survive the hardships and find the strength to keep going? After my personal ordeal, I couldn't help feeling it was a race I was suited for.

Before the '99 season began, I went to Indianapolis for a cancer-awareness dinner, and I stopped by the hospital to see my old cancer friends. Scott Shapiro said, "So, you're returning to stage racing?"

I said yes, and then I asked a question. "Do you think I can win the Tour de France?"

"I not only think you can," he said. "I expect you to."

BUT I KEPT CRASHING.

At first, the 1999 cycling season was a total failure. In the second race of the year, the Tour of Valencia, I crashed off the bike and almost broke my shoulder. I took two weeks off, but no sooner did I get back on than I crashed again: I was on a training ride in the south of France when an elderly woman ran her car off the side of the road and sideswiped me. I suffered like the proverbial dog through Paris–Nice and Milan–San Remo in lousy weather, struggling to mid-pack finishes. I wrote it off to early-season bad form, and went on to the next race—where I crashed again. On the last corner of the first stage, I spun out in the rain. My tires went out from under me in a dusky oil slick and I tumbled off the bike.

I went home. The problem was simply that I was rusty, so for two solid weeks I worked on my technique, until I felt secure in the saddle. When I came back, I stayed upright. I finally won something, a time-trial stage in the Circuit de la Sarthe. My results picked up.

But it was funny, I wasn't as good in the one-day races anymore. I was no longer the angry and unsettled young rider I had been. My racing was still intense, but it had become subtler in style and technique, not as visibly aggressive. Something different fueled me now—psychologically, physically, and emotionally—and that something was the Tour de France.

I was willing to sacrifice the entire season to prepare for the Tour. I staked everything on it. I skipped all the spring classics, the prestigious races that comprised the backbone of the international cycling tour, and instead picked and chose only a handful of events that would help me peak in July. Nobody could understand what I was doing. In the past, I'd made my living in the classics. Why wasn't I riding in the races

I'd won before? Finally a journalist came up to me and asked if I was entered in any of the spring classics.

"No," I said.

"Well, why not?"

"I'm focusing on the Tour."

He kind of smirked at me and said, "Oh, so you're a Tour rider now." Like I was joking.

I just looked at him, and thought, *Whatever, dude. We'll see.*

Not long afterward, I ran into Miguel Indurain in a hotel elevator. He, too, asked me what I was doing.

"I'm spending a lot of time training in the Pyrenees," I said.

"Porque?" he asked "Why?"

"For the Tour," I said.

He lifted an eyebrow in surprise, and reserved comment.

Every member of our Postal team was as committed to the Tour as I was. The Postal roster was as follows: Frankie Andreu was a big, powerful sprinter and our captain, an accomplished veteran who had known me since I was a teenager. Kevin Livingston and Tyler Hamilton were our talented young climbing specialists; George Hincapie was the U.S. Pro champion and another rangy sprinter like Frankie; Christian Vandevelde was one of the most talented rookies around; Pascal Derame, Jonathan Vaughters, and Peter Meinert-Neilsen were loyal domestiques who would ride at high speed for hours without complaint.

The man who shaped us into a team was our director, Johan Bruyneel, a poker-faced Belgian and former Tour rider. Johan knew what was required to win the Tour; he had won stages twice during his own career. In 1993, he won what at the time was the fastest stage in Tour history, and in 1995, he won another when he outdueled Indurain in a spectacular finish into Liège. It was just Johan and Indurain alone at the front, and he sat on Indurain's wheel the whole way, until he pulled around and beat him in the sprint across the line. He was a smart, resourceful rider who knew how to beat more powerful competitors, and he brought the same sure sense of strategy to our team.

It was Johan's idea to hold training camps. We bought into his plan, refusing to complain, and spent a week apiece in the Alps and the Pyrenees. We scouted the mountain terrain of the Tour, and practiced the climbs we'd be facing, riding back-to-back seven-hour days in all weather. As we went over the mountainous sections, I worked especially closely with Kevin and Tyler because they were our climbers, the guys who would have to do most of the work pulling me up those gradients. While most other riders were resting in the off-season or competing in the classics, we rode uphill in foul conditions.

Johan and I had a running joke. It was January in the Pyrenees, and every day it pissed down rain. I was getting beat up, hammered by those climbs, while Johan followed in the warmth of a car, talking me through it via a two-way radio.

One day I got on the air and said, "Johan."

"Yes, Lance, what do you want?"

"I'm doing the classics next year."

From then on, I said it every day. Pretty soon Johan knew what was coming.

"Johan."

"Let me guess, Lance," he'd say, tonelessly. "You're doing the classics next year."

"Right."

When we weren't in the Alps or Pyrenees, I trained on my own. There was a purpose to everything I did. Kik and I lived day in and day out with only two things in mind: the Tour de France and having a healthy baby. Anything else was secondary, an unnecessary distraction. But there was a sort of peace in the simplicity of our dedication.

I geeked out. I tackled the problem of the Tour as if I were in math class, science class, chemistry class, and nutrition class, all rolled into one. I did computer calculations that balanced my body weight and my equipment weight with the potential velocity of the bike in various stages, trying to find the equation that would get me to the finish line faster than anybody else. I kept careful computer graphs of my training rides, calibrating the distances, wattages, and thresholds.

Even eating became mathematical. I measured my food intake. I kept a small scale in the kitchen and weighed the portions of pasta and bread. Then I calculated my wattages versus my caloric intake, so I knew precisely how much to eat each day, how many calories to burn, so that the amount coming in would be less than my output, and I would lose weight.

There was one unforeseen benefit of cancer: it had completely re-shaped my body. I now had a much sparer build. In old pictures, I looked like a football player with my thick neck and big upper body, which had contributed to my bullishness on the bike. But paradoxi-cally, my strength had held me back in the mountains, because it took so much work to haul that weight uphill. Now I was almost gaunt, and the result was a lightness I'd never felt on the bike before. I was leaner in body and more balanced in spirit.

The doubt about me as a Tour rider was my climbing ability. I could always sprint, but the mountains were my downfall. Eddy Merckx had been telling me to slim down for years, and now I un-derstood why. A five-pound drop was a large weight loss for the moun-tains—and I had lost 15 pounds. It was all I needed. I became very good in the mountains.

Each morning I rose and ate the same thing for breakfast, some muesli with bread and fruit, unless it was going to be a particularly long training ride, in which case I had a plate of scrambled egg whites. While I ate, Kik filled my water bottles, and I bolted out the door by 8 A.M. to join Kevin and Tyler for a training ride. Most days I would ride straight through lunch, until about 3 P.M. When I came home I'd shower and lie down for a nap until dinnertime. I'd get up again in the evening, weigh my pasta, and have dinner with Kik.

We didn't do anything. We didn't go anywhere. We just ate, and then went back to bed, so I could get up in the morning and train again. That was our life for several months. Sometimes Kik's friends would say, "Oh, you live in the South of France, how glamorous." They had no idea.

While I trained, Kik would do errands or rest on our veranda. She thought Nice was the perfect place to be pregnant, because she could wander the outdoor markets buying fresh fruit and vegetables. In the evenings we would thumb through pregnancy books and follow the growth of the baby. First it was the size of a pin, then a lemon. The big day came when Kik had trouble buttoning her jeans for the first time.

The extent of the commitment from Kik as well as from me was very serious. Cycling was a hard, hard job, and Kik respected it as such. "Have a good day at work," she said each morning as I left. If we both hadn't been equally dedicated to the lifestyle, it wouldn't have worked. If she had felt bored, cheated, or discontented, we could not have gotten through the months peacefully. She might as well have been a team domestique, that's how integral she was to my training process.

Kevin could see it, because he was our best friend and also had an apartment in Nice. Unlike me, he had no one to come home to in Europe. When he returned from a race or training camp he came back to an empty apartment, and sometimes to spoiled milk. I had fresh laundry, a clean house, a cat, a dog, and everything I needed to eat. But it took a lot of work from Kik to keep it up. I had always been uncomfortable and lonesome living in Europe, until I did it as a happily married man. Now I was learning to love it.

There were days when I had a flat and was out in the middle of nowhere, and I'd call home and Kik would come look for me. Some afternoons she would drive up into the mountains just to bring me Gatorade and food. She learned everything about cycling, so she could be helpful. She knew what I needed and when, which days were the tough ones, when it was good to talk, and when to leave me alone.

On the really hard training days, she would be on pins and needles waiting to see how it had gone, because she knew how I measured my preparation and how important it was for me to be on target. If it didn't go well, she understood my disappointment and my grumpiness.

At the end of April, I returned to racing in a prestigious one-day classic called the Amstel Gold Race, to gauge my form. From the start, I felt like a different, stronger rider. For much of the day I dueled with Michael Boogerd of Holland, considered one of the top riders in the world.

With ten miles to go, I rode at the front. Boogerd sat on my wheel, trailing me. By now I knew, or at least I thought I knew, that I was going to beat him in the final sprint to the finish. I would have bet my health on it. I was that certain.

I started the last sprint—and Boogerd came out of the box. He cut around and drew even with me, and we dashed the last few hundred yards—and I lost. I lost by a centimeter. Less than a tire width.

I was devastated. I had been absolutely certain I would win, but what cut me the most was that Boogerd was widely considered a big favorite to win the Tour de France. As we stood side by side on the podium, all I could think about was what it meant for my Tour plans. Suddenly, I leaned over and I said to Michael, "You're going to pay me back in July."

He looked at me strangely. "What are you talking about?" he said. "It's April."

I went back to training. I rode, and I rode, and I rode. I rode like I had never ridden, punishing my body up and down every hill I could find. There were something like 50 good, arduous climbs around Nice, solid inclines of ten miles or more. The trick was not to climb every once in a while, but to climb repeatedly. I would do three different climbs in a day, over the course of a six- or seven-hour ride. A 12-mile climb took about an hour, so that tells you what my days were like.

I rode when no one else would ride, sometimes not even my team-mates. I remember one day in particular, May 3, a raw European spring day, biting cold. I steered my bike into the Alps, with Johan following in a car. By now it was sleeting and 32 degrees. I didn't care. We stood at the roadside and looked at the view and the weather, and Johan suggested that we skip it. I said, "No. Let's do it." I rode for seven straight hours, alone. To win the Tour I had to be willing to ride when no one else would ride.

The most punishing ride in Nice was the Col de la Madone, or the Madonna. It was a famously tough eight-mile climb above the city. You could almost see it from our house, beyond the rolling hills that ringed the skyline. The Madone was too difficult to train on all the time, but it was a great test of fitness. Most people did it once or twice in a season. I did it once a month.

Tony Rominger, who for years was one of the top riders in the world, used the Madone as his training test when he lived in Monaco, and he held the record for climbing it—31 minutes and 30 seconds. Kevin Livingston, arguably the best climber on our Postal Service team, once did it in 32 minutes. At the beginning of my comeback in the '98 season, I had done the Madone in 36 minutes. But to win the Tour, I knew I had to whittle the time down considerably.

"I'm going to break 31," I announced to Kevin one day.

That was big talk coming from someone who at the time couldn't even break 35 on the hill.

"You're crazy," Kevin said.

But I got to 34, and then 33. Then one afternoon, I clocked in at

32:30. Right before the Tour, Kevin and I rode the Madone one last time.

It was a humid day, with just a little bit of wind, very muggy and hot. We raced toward the peak, which was in clouds, 3,000 feet above sea level. With a kilometer to go, Kevin flatted. While he stopped to change his tire, I pedaled on. As I got to the top, I glanced at the time clock on my handlebars.

I waited for Kevin. He arrived out of breath and in a bad mood over his flat tire. I showed him the time on my computer. The implications for the Tour hit us. "Oh, boy," Kevin said. "This could be ugly."

Kik knew that whenever I did the Madone, it was a serious day. I had been stone-faced over breakfast, already concentrating. When I came home she was waiting by the front door, anxious to see how it had gone, whether I was cheerful or testy. Och was visiting us, and he waited anxiously, too.

I barged into the house, looking grim.

"How'd it go?" she asked.

"The conditions were lousy," I said.

"Oh," she said.

"Yeah," I said. "All I did was a 30:47."

She threw her arms around me. Och slapped me on the back.

"Jimmy, I'm ready," I said.

A few days later, Och went back to the States. He told everybody who would listen that I was going to win the Tour de France.

I PACKED FOR THE TOUR WITH A COMPULSIVE, NERVOUS attention to detail. Kik and I laid out all my things and arranged them carefully in the suitcase. I insisted they be packed a certain way. My bike shorts had to be rolled together so that they fit in a neat line. My shoeboxes had to be set in the right place. Gloves were tucked into a particular corner, arm warmers into another. Everything had to be perfectly aligned, so I knew at a glance that I had every type of clothing for every type of weather.

We arrived in Paris for the preliminaries to the Tour, which included a series of medical and drug tests, and mandatory lectures from Tour officials. Each rider was given a Tour "Bible," a guidebook that showed every stage of the course, with profiles of the route and where the feed areas were. We tinkered with our bikes, changing handlebars and making sure our cleats fit the pedals just right. Some riders were more casual than others about the setup of their bikes, but I was particular. The crew called me Mister Millimeter.

In the prerace hype, our U.S. Postal team was considered an outside shot. No one talked about us as having a chance of winning. They talked about Abraham Olano, the reigning world champion. They talked about Michael Boogerd, who had beaten me in the Amstel. They talked about Alexander Zulle of Switzerland and Fernando Escartin of Spain. They talked about who wasn't there, the casualties of the doping investigations. I was a footnote, the heartwarming American cancer survivor. Only one person seemed to think I was capable of it. Shortly before the race began, someone asked Miguel Indurain who he thought had a good chance of winning. Maybe he remembered our conversation in the elevator and knew how I had trained. "Armstrong" was his answer.

The first stage of the Tour was the brief Prologue, a time trial of eight kilometers in Le Puy du Fou, a town with a parchment-colored chateau and a medieval theme park. The Prologue was a seeding system of sorts, to separate out the fast riders from the slow and determine who would ride at the front of the peloton. Although it was only eight kilometers long, it was a serious test with absolutely no margin for error. You had to sprint flat-out, and find maximum efficiency, or you would be behind before you ever started. The riders who wanted to contend in the overall needed to finish among the top three or four.

The course began with a sprint of five kilometers, and then came a big hill, a long suffer-fest of 700 meters—a climb you couldn't afford to do at anything less than all-out. After a sweeping turn, it was a flat sprint to the finish. The course would favor a bullish rider like me, and it had also been perfect for the great Indurain, who had once ridden it in a record time of 8:12.

All told, it should take less than nine minutes. The biggest factor was the hill. You didn't want to spend all your energy in the first 5K sprint, and then die on the hill. Also, there was a strategic decision to be made: should I take the hill with a big chainring, or a smaller one? We debated the matter on and off for two days.

Johan was calm and exacting as he plotted our strategy. He broke the race down into wattages and split times, and gave me precise instructions. He even knew what my heart rate should be over the first sprint: 190.

Riders went off in staggered starts three minutes apart. Reports drifted back from the course. Frankie Andreu, my teammate, sacrificed himself with an experiment when he tried to climb the hill using the big ring. It was the wrong decision. By the time he reached the top of the hill, he was done, blown. He never recovered.

Olano broke the course record with a time of 8:11. Then Zulle beat that with an 8:07.

It was my turn. When I'm riding well, my body seems almost motionless on the bike with the exception of my legs, which look like automated pistons. From behind in the team car, Johan could see that my shoulders barely swayed, meaning I was wasting no extra energy, everything was going into the bike, pumping it down the road.

In my ear, Johan gave me partial time checks and instructions as I rode.

"You're out of the saddle," Johan said. "Sit down."

I was pushing too hard, not realizing it. I sat down, and focused on execution, on the science and technique of the ride. I had no idea what my overall time was. I just pedaled.

I crossed the finish line. I glanced at the clock.

It read "8:02."

I thought, *That can't be right.*

I looked again. "8:02."

I was the leader of the Tour de France. For the first time in my career, I would wear the yellow jersey, the *maillot jaune,* to distinguish me from the other riders.

At our campers, I got giant bear hugs from my teammates, and the biggest of all from Johan. An ESPN camera crew arrived for an interview, but I could barely get through it. My mouth felt tight, and I was afraid I would break down on the air. I couldn't talk. I couldn't get the words out. "I'm just in shock," I said, hoarsely. "I'm in shock."

Out of the crowd, I saw Indurain. He pushed through and came toward me, and gave me an affectionate handshake and hug.

There is really no time to celebrate a stage win in the Tour. First you're hustled to drug testing, and then protocol takes over. I was ushered to a camper to wash up for the podium ceremony, and presented with the yellow jersey to change into. As much as I had prepared for the Tour, this moment was the one thing I had left out. I hadn't prepared for the sensation of pulling on that jersey, of feeling the fabric slide over my back.

Back home in Nice, Kik watched on TV as I stepped onto the podium in the yellow jersey. She jumped around our house, shrieking and shaking up the baby, and making the dog bark. Finally, I got down from the podium and went into our team camper, where I used the phone to call her. "Babe," I said.

All I heard on the other end of the line was, "Oh my God, oh my

God, oh my God!" and she burst into tears. Then she said, "Damn, honey, you did it."

There was a second supremely sweet moment of victory. As I made my way through the finish area, I passed the Cofidis team. Assorted members of the organization stood around, the men who I felt had left me for dead in a hospital room.

"That was for you," I said, as I moved past them.

WE SET OFF ACROSS THE NORTHERN PLAINS OF FRANCE. I was the first American riding for an American team, on an American bike, ever to lead the Tour de France. That morning, I looked at the date: it was July 4.

Suddenly, I got nervous. The yellow jersey was a responsibility. Now, instead of being the attacker, I would be the rider under attack. I had never been in the position of defending the jersey before.

The opening stages of the Tour were the terrain of sprinters. We hurtled across the plains on flat and monotonous roads, playing our game of speed chess on bikes. Nerves were taut; there was a lot of maneuvering and flicking in the peloton, close calls, and a couple of classic Tour crashes.

Handlebars clashed, hips bumped, tires collided. There was less to contend with at the front of the peloton, so that's where we tried to ride, but so did every other team, and the road was only so wide. With almost 200 riders jockeying for position, it was tough to avoid collisions. The main strategy in those first few days was to stay out of trouble—easier said than done. In the position battle, with such constant movement, you could get spit out the back before you knew it. The year before, Kevin had crashed twice in the flats and found himself 15 minutes down before he ever reached the mountains.

Our team setup consisted of two following cars and a van. In one car were Johan and the crew, with our reserve bikes on top, and in the other were team managers and any sponsors who happened to be along for the ride. The van carried all the bikes and our bags and assorted other equipment. If someone got a flat tire, a mechanic was available, and if we needed water or food, the crew could hand it to us.

Johan directed the race tactically from the car. He issued time checks and status reports and attack orders over a sophisticated two-way radio system. Each Postal rider had an earpiece and a small black radio cord around his collar, and was wired with a heart monitor so that Johan could keep track of how our bodies were performing under stress.

All day, every day, my teammates rode in front of me, protecting me from wind, crashes, competitors, and other hazards. We constantly dodged overeager spectators and photographers and their various paraphernalia: baby carriages, coolers, you name it.

In the second stage, we came to a four-kilometer causeway called the Passage du Gois, a scene of almost surreal strangeness. The Passage is a long, narrow, blacktop road across a tidal marsh, but the brackish water floods at high tide, covering the road and making it impassable. Even when the road is passable, it's slick and treacherous, and the edges are covered with barnacles and seaweed.

The peloton was still bunched up, full of banging and maneuvering, and it would be a tricky crossing. The first teams across would have the safest passage, so most of the Postal riders gathered around me and we surged near the front. Along the way, some of our teammates got separated and wound up in a second group. Frankie and George got me over with no mishaps, but it was frightening; the road was so slippery under our tires that we hesitated to so much as turn the wheel, and we fought a crosswind that made it hard to keep the bike straight.

Behind us, other riders weren't so lucky. They rode straight into a massive pileup.

Somebody hit his brakes, and suddenly there were competitors lying all over the blacktop. Bikes flew up in the air, wheels spinning crazily, and riders tumbled to the ground in a huge chain reaction. Guys lay prone on the asphalt as the rest of the peloton bore down on them, and more riders fell. We lost Jonathan Vaughters, who banged his head and cut his chin wide open, and had to abandon. Jonathan had averted disaster the previous day in another crash, when he vaulted headfirst over his handlebars—and managed to land on his feet. He earned the nickname of El Gato, "The Cat," from the peloton for that, but now he was out. Tyler Hamilton came away from the crash with a sore knee.

As it turned out, the Passage du Gois was one of the more critical moments of the race. By getting across the Passage early, I picked up valuable time, while some of those bodies scattered behind me in the road were Tour favorites. Michael Boogerd and Alex Zulle fell more than six minutes behind—a deficit that would become more and more telling as the days wore on.

Over those first ten days, we had just one aim—to stay near the front and out of any more trouble. I was seeking a balance: I wanted to remain in contention, while staying as fresh as possible for the more crucial upcoming stage, a time trial in Metz. I gave up the yellow jersey for the time being.

These were some of the longest days of the Tour, and there was a sameness to the roads and scenery. We went from Nantes to Laval, to Amiens, but it seemed like we rode forever without going anywhere. Mario Cippolini of Italy won four consecutive stages to tie a Tour record, and we conceded them without a fight. Cippolini was a great rider, but he wasn't a climber and we all knew he wouldn't be a factor for the overall victory.

Each night we shared the same routine: massages for our sore legs, dinner, and then we would surf the six channels of French TV available in the hotel. Johan banned me from bringing my computer, because I had a tendency to stay up too late fooling around online.

We sped on, across the plains, toward Metz.

I hung back, saving myself.

It is called the Race of Truth. The early stages separate the strong riders from the weak. Now the weak would be eliminated altogether.

We arrived in Metz for the time trial, and in this one, unlike the brief Prologue, riders would have an opportunity to win or lose big chunks of time. It was 56 kilometers long, which meant riding full-out for more than an hour, and those riders who didn't make the time cut were gone, out of the race. Hence the phrase "Race of Truth."

Kik came in from Nice. For much of the first week she had watched us on television at home, but she would spend the rest of the Tour traveling in Europe with her parents to keep the boredom and tension at bay, while checking in with me periodically. The Tour wasn't exactly the ideal situation for a conjugal visit, because I was sequestered with the team, but seeing her for a day was better than nothing, and I got to check on how her pregnancy was progressing. Also, having her in Metz reminded me of how hard I had worked and studied for this occasion.

Early in the morning of the stage, I went out and previewed the course, but I was already familiar with it, because we had scouted it during training camp. It had two very big climbs, one 1.5K long and the other 4K long. The early part would be windy, then came the hills, and the final flats would be into a strong headwind. It was a course that favored strength, a rider who could drive a big gear into the teeth of that wind. It wasn't enough to be fast; I would have to be fast for over an hour.

As I warmed up on a stationary bike, results filtered in. The riders went out in staggered fashion, two minutes apart, and Alex Zulle, the Swiss favorite who had suffered the unfortunate crash on the Passage du Gois, was the early leader with a time of a little over an hour and nine minutes. I wasn't surprised; Zulle was a strapping blond strongman without an ounce of give-up, as I would continue to learn throughout the race.

The pre-race favorite, Abraham Olano, set off on the course just in front of me. But as I waited in the start area, word came through that Olano had crashed on a small curve, losing about 30 seconds. He got back on his bike, but his rhythm was gone.

My turn. I went out hard—maybe too hard. In my ear, Johan kept up his usual stream of steady advice and information. At the first two checkpoints, he reported, I had the fastest splits.

Third checkpoint: I was ahead of Zulle by a minute and forty seconds.

Ahead of me, I saw Olano.

Olano had never been caught in a time trial, and now he began glancing over his shoulder. I jackhammered at my pedals.

I was on top of him. The look on Olano's face was incredulous, and dismayed. I caught him—and passed him. He disappeared behind my back wheel.

Johan talked into my ear. My cadence was up at 100 rpms. "That's high," Johan warned. I was pedaling too hard. I eased off.

I swept into a broad downhill turn, with hay bales packed by the side of the road. Now I saw another figure ahead of me. A rider was lying by the side of the road, injured and waiting for medical attention. I recognized the colors of the Cofidis team.

Bobby Julich.

He had lost control and skidded out on the turn. I would learn later that he had badly bruised his chest and ribs. His race was over.

I went into a tuck around the turn.

From out of the crowd, a child ran into the road.

I swerved wide to avoid him, my heart pounding.

Quickly, I regained my composure and never broke rhythm. Ahead of me, I saw yet another rider. I squinted, trying to make out who it was, and saw a flash of green. It was the jersey of Tom Steels of Belgium, a superb sprinter who'd won two of the flat early stages, and who was a contender for the overall title.

But Steels had started six minutes in front of me. Had I ridden that fast?

Johan, normally so controlled and impassive, checked the time. He began screaming into the radio.

"You're blowing up the Tour de France!" he howled. "You're blowing up the Tour de France!"

I passed Steels.

I could feel the lactic acid seeping through my legs. My face was one big grimace of pain. I had gone out too hard—and now I was paying. I entered the last stretch, into that headwind, and I felt as though I could barely move. With each rotation of my wheels, I gave time back to Zulle. The seconds ticked by as I labored toward the finish.

Finally, I crossed the line.

I checked the clock: 1:08:36. I was the winner. I had beaten Zulle by 58 seconds.

I fell off the bike, so tired I was cross-eyed. As tired as I have ever been. But I led the Tour de France again. As I pulled the yellow jersey over my head, and once more felt the smooth fabric slide over my back, I decided that's where it needed to stay.

I stepped down off the podium and handed Kik the flowers, and gave her a huge hug and a kiss. That evening, I told her, "I think I'm going to win this thing."

Back at the team hotel, we Postal riders drank a glass of Champagne together. We only sipped it, because the day's ride had taken so much out of us that a glass felt like a whole bottle. After we completed the toast, Johan stood up.

"Okay, no more Champagne," he said. "That's the last time we drink it, because we're going to win so many stages that we'd drink it all the way to Paris."

The team cheered.

WE ENTERED THE MOUNTAINS.

From now on, everything would be uphill, including the finish lines. The first Alpine stage was a ride of 132.7 kilometers into the chalet-studded town of Sestrière, on the French–Italian border, and I knew what the peloton was thinking: that I would fold. They didn't respect the yellow jersey on my back.

I held a lead of two minutes and 20 seconds, but in the mountains you could fall hopelessly behind in a single day. I had never been a renowned climber, and now we were about to embark on the most grueling and storied stages of the race, through peaks that made riders crack like walnuts. I was sure to come under heavy attack from my adversaries, but what they didn't know was how specifically and hard I had trained for this part of the race. It was time to show them.

It would be a tactical ride as much as a physical one, and I would have to rely heavily on my fellow climbers, Kevin Livingston and Tyler Hamilton. Drafting is hugely important in the mountains: Kevin and Tyler would do much of the grueling work of riding uphill in front of me, so I could conserve my energy for the last big climb into Sestriere, where the other riders were sure to try to grab the jersey from me.

Here's how an "attack" works: some riders were more threatening than others, like Alex Zulle of Switzerland and Fernando Escartin of

Spain, the men who trailed me most closely throughout the race. If one of them, say Zulle, tried to break away, one of my Postal teammates, let's say Kevin, immediately chased him down. A rider like Zulle could get away and be two minutes up the road before we knew it, and cut into my overall lead.

Kevin's job was to get behind Zulle and stay right behind his wheel, making it harder for Zulle to pull up the hill. It's called "sitting on him." While Kevin "sat" on Zulle's wheel and slowed him down, the rest of my Postal teammates pulled me, riding in front of me, allowing me to draft and catch up. If we could get through the day without succumbing to any major attacks, it was called "managing the peloton" or "controlling" it.

We didn't chase down every breakaway. Some riders were not a threat to the overall title, and we didn't waste our energy chasing them down. At those times, my teammates just took care of me. They surrounded me and made sure I was positioned safe from harm. If I needed a new water bottle, one of them went back to the team car and got it for me.

There were three big cols, or peaks, en route to Sestriere. The first was the Col du Télégraphe, then came the monstrous Col du Galibier, the tallest mountain in the Tour, then Col de Montgenèvre. Lastly, there would be the uphill finish into Sestrière.

For the better part of 150 miles that day, Postal was a machine, making seamless transitions and controlling the action.

The Spanish attacked us right from the start. Escartin launched a breakaway on the Télégraphe in a kind of sucker play, but we kept calm and refused to expend too much energy too early. On the Galibier, Kevin Livingston did magnificent work, pulling me steadily to the top, where it was sleeting and hailing. As I drafted behind Kevin, I kept up a stream of encouragement. "You're doing great, man," I said. "These guys behind us are dying."

We descended the Galibier in sweeping curves through the pines. Let me describe that descent to you. You hunch over your handlebars and streak seventy miles an hour on two small tires a half-inch wide, shivering. Now throw in curves, switchbacks, hairpins, and fog. Water streamed down the mountainside under my wheels, and somewhere behind me, Kevin crashed. He had tried to put on a rain jacket, and the sleeve got caught in his wheel. He recovered, but he would be sore and feverish for the next few days.

Now came Montgenèvre, our third mountain ascent in the space of six hours, into more freezing rains and mist. We would ride into a rain shower, then out the other side. At the peak it was so cold, the rain froze to my shirt. On the descent, it hailed. Now I was separated from the rest of the team, and the attacks kept coming, as if the other riders thought I was going to crack at any moment. It made me angry. The weaker riders fell away, unable to keep up. I found myself out in front among the top climbers in the world, working alone. I intended to make them suffer until they couldn't breathe.

All I had for company was the sound of Johan's voice in my ear. He was in the follow car. Riding shotgun was Thom Weisel, the chief patron of the team.

On the descent from Montgenèvre, Ivan Gotti and Fernando Escartin gambled on the hairpin turns through the mists, and opened up a gap of 25 seconds. I trailed them in a second group of five cyclists.

We went into the final ascent, the long, hard 30K climb into Sestrière itself. We had been on the bikes for five and a half hours, and all of us were struggling. From here on in it would be a question of who cracked and who didn't.

With eight kilometers to go, I was 32 seconds behind the leaders, and locked in the second group of five riders, all of us churning uphill. The others were all established climbers of various nationality, the best of them Zulle of Switzerland, burly and indefatigable and haunting me.

It was time to go.

On a small curve, I swung to the inside of the group, stood up, and accelerated. My bike seemed to jump ahead. I almost rode up the backs of the escort motorcycles.

From the follow car, a surprised Johan said, "Lance, you've got a gap." Then he said, "Ten feet."

Johan checked my heart rate via the digital computer readout, so he knew how hard I was working and how stressed my body was. I was at 180, not in distress. I felt as though I was just cruising along a flat road, riding comfortably.

He said, "Lance, the gap's getting bigger."

I ripped across the space.

In one kilometer I made up 21 seconds. I was now just 11 seconds back of the leaders. It was strange, but I still didn't feel a thing. It was . . . *effortless.*

The two front-runners, Escartin and Gotti, were looking over their shoulders. I continued to close rapidly.

I rode up to Escartin's back wheel. He glanced back at me, incredulous. Gotti tried to pick up the pace. I accelerated past him, and drew even with Escartin.

I surged again, driving the pace just a little higher. I was probing, seeking information on their fitness and states of mind, how they would respond.

I opened a tiny gap, curious. Were they tired?

No response.

"One length," Johan said.

I accelerated.

"Three lengths, four lengths, five lengths."

Johan paused. Then he said, almost casually, "Why don't you put a little more on?"

I accelerated again.

"Forty feet," he said.

When you open a gap, and your competitors don't respond, it tells you something. They're hurting. And when they're hurting, that's when you take them.

We were four miles from the finish. I drove my legs down onto the pedals.

"You've got thirty seconds!" Johan said, more excitedly.

In my ear, Johan continued to narrate my progress. Now he reported that Zulle was trying to chase. Zulle, always Zulle.

"Look, I'm just going to go," I said into my radio. "I'm going to put this thing away."

IN A HOTEL ROOM IN ITALY, KIK SAT TRANSFIXED IN front of the TV. As I jumped out of my seat and charged, she leaped up out of her chair.

"Haul ass!" she yelled.

In Plano, Texas, later that day, my mother would watch a tape delay of the stage. Because of the time change, she didn't yet know what had happened.

"Look out!" she yelled. "There he goes! He's got it!"

THE BIKE SWAYED UNDER ME AS I WORKED THE PEDALS, and my shoulders began heaving with fatigue. I felt a creeping exhaustion, and my body was moving all over the top of the bike. My nostrils flared, as I struggled to breathe, fighting for any extra air at all. I bared my teeth in a half-snarl.

It was still a long haul to the finish, and I was concerned Zulle would catch me. But I maintained my rhythm.

I glanced over my shoulder, half expecting to see Zulle on my wheel.

No one was there.

I faced forward again. Now I could see the finish line—it was all uphill the rest of the way. I drove toward the peak.

Was I thinking of cancer as I rode those last few hundred yards? No. I'd be lying if I said I was. But I think that directly or indirectly, what had happened over the past two years was with me. It was stacked up and stored away, everything I'd been through, the bout with cancer, and the disbelief within the sport that I could come back. It either made me faster or them slower, I don't know which.

As I continued to climb, I felt pain, but I felt exultation, too, at what I could do with my body. To race and suffer, that's hard. But it's not being laid out in a hospital bed with a catheter hanging out of your chest, platinum burning in your veins, throwing up for 24 hours straight, five days a week.

What was I thinking? A funny thing. I remembered a scene in *Good Will Hunting,* a movie in which Matt Damon plays an alienated young math prodigy, an angry kid from the wrong side of the South Boston tracks, not unlike me. In the film he tries to socialize with some upper-class Harvard students in a bar, and wins a duel of wits with a pompous intellectual to win a girl's affections.

Afterward Damon gloats to the guy he bested, "Hey. Do you like apples?"

"Yeah," the guy says, "I like apples."

"Well, I got her phone number," Damon says triumphantly. "How do you like them apples?"

I climbed those hundreds of meters, sucking in the thin mountain air, and I thought of that movie, and grinned.

As I approached the finish line, I spoke into my radio to my friends in the support car, Johan and Thom Weisel.

"Hey, Thom, Johan," I said. "Do you like apples?"

Their puzzled reply crackled in my ear.

"Yeah, we like apples. Why?"

I yelled into the mouthpiece, *"How do you like them fuckin' apples!"*

I hit the finish line with my arms upraised, my eyes toward the sky. And then I put my hands to my face in disbelief.

IN HER HOTEL ROOM IN ITALY, MY WIFE SAT IN FRONT of the television, sobbing.

Later that day in Indianapolis, LaTrice Haney and the staff of the medical center, and all of the patients on the ward, stopped what they were doing to watch the taped coverage. As I mounted the hill, increasing my lead, they stared at their televisions. "He did it," LaTrice said. "He conquered it. He conquered it."

With the climb into Sestrière I now led the Tour de France by six minutes, three seconds.

YOU DON'T REALLY SEE THE MOUNTAINS AS YOU RIDE through them. There is no time to dwell on the view, on the majestic cliffs and precipices and shelves that rise on either side of you, looming rock with glaciers and peaks, falling away into green pastures. All you really notice is the road in front of you, and the riders in back of you, because no lead is safe in the mountains.

On the morning after Sestrière I rose early and had breakfast with the team. We went through 25 boxes of cereal each week, and dozens and dozens of eggs. First I powered down some muesli, then a plate of three or four eggs, and after that I shoveled in some pasta. It would be another long, hard climbing day, and I needed every ounce of carbo-driven energy I could find. We would be riding the Alpe d'Huez, a stage that held as much mystique as any in the Tour, a 1,000-meter climb over 14 kilometers, with a nine-degree gradient. The ascent included 21 tortuous hairpin turns, a seemingly endless series of switch-backs leading to the summit. It was hot going up and cold coming down, and in some places the road was only as wide as my handlebars. Back in the early 1900s, when the mountain climbs were added to the Tour for the first time, one rider completed the journey up on his ponderous old contraption, and then turned to race organizers at the roadside and screamed, "You're all murderers!"

I wanted to avoid any high drama on the Alpe d'Huez. I didn't need to attack as I had at Sestrière, I simply needed to keep my chief opponents in check: Abraham Olano was six minutes and three seconds behind me, and Alex Zulle was in fourth place, trailing by seven minutes, 47 seconds. Fernando Escartin was in eighth place, down by nine minutes. The goal for the day was to be steady and not to give back any of the time I had gained at Sestrière.

We reached the base of the Alpe d'Huez. I wanted to let the team know I was in good shape, because morale was critical on a tough climb. Everybody had an earpiece and access to the two-way radio, so I knew they could all hear me.

"Hey, Johan," I said.

"Yes, Lance," he said, in that monotone.

"I could do this thing on a damn tricycle. It's not a problem."

I could hear cackling in the background.

We rode at a fast tempo, to limit the attacks and whittle down the riders who could challenge us. First, Tyler Hamilton pulled me up the mountain. I sat on his wheel and talked to him the whole way, right into his ear. We moved past Olano. Johan came over the radio, reporting, "Olano is dropped. Great job." Here came Manuel Beltran, one of Zulle's teammates. I yelled at Tyler. "Are you going to let Beltran do that to you?"

We had 10K to go, about 30 minutes of work, straight uphill. Suddenly, here came Escartin and his teammate, Carlos Contreras, accelerating into the climb. Then Pavel Tonkov, a teammate of Tom Steels, launched an attack. Tyler was done. He had nothing left, so I had to chase down Tonkov myself. Then came Zulle, with Beltran pulling him, while the French climber, Richard Virenque, came up and sat on my wheel. They were all trying to put me on the ropes.

But I wasn't tiring. All of this action was fine by me, because as long as I stayed with them no one could make up any significant time on me. I continued along in fourth place, keeping an eye on everything. We had 4K to go to reach the summit, about six and a half more minutes of duress. An Italian, Giuseppe Guerini, a decorated rider who had twice finished third in the Tour of Italy, charged. But Guerini was 15 minutes down in the overall standings, and I didn't need to counter him. I let him go. Meanwhile, Zulle finally cracked. He couldn't keep the pace.

Guerini opened up a 20-second lead—and then, unbelievably, he hit a spectator. The spectators had been flirting with disaster for days, skipping across the road in front of the peloton, and now a frenzied fan had leaped into the middle of the road with his Instamatic, and stood there taking pictures. Guerini moved one way and then the other, trying to avoid him, but plowed right into him with the handlebars, and went over. It was a classic Tour moment, proof that no lead was safe. Guerini jumped up unhurt and continued on, but now Tonkov was breathing on him. Fortunately, Guerini got over the line first, the stage winner.

I finished the stage in fifth place. I now had a lead of 7:42 over Olano in the overall. Zulle, for all his work, had made up only seconds, and trailed by 7:47.

Just a typical day in the Tour de France.

I WAS MAKING ENEMIES IN THE ALPS. MY NEWLY AC-quired climbing prowess aroused suspicion in the French press, still sniffing for blood after the scandal of the previous summer. A whispering campaign began: "Armstrong must be on something." Stories in *L'Equipe* and *Le Monde* insinuated, without saying it outright, that my comeback was a little too miraculous.

I knew there would be consequences for Sestrière—it was almost a tradition that any rider who wore the yellow jersey was subject to drug speculation. But I was taken aback by the improbable nature of the charges in the French press: some reporters actually suggested that chemotherapy had been beneficial to my racing. They speculated that I had been given some mysterious drug during the treatments that was performance-enhancing. Any oncologist in the world, regardless of nationality, had to laugh himself silly at the suggestion.

I didn't understand it. How could anybody think for a second that somehow the cancer treatments had helped me? Maybe no one but a cancer patient understands the severity of the treatment. For three straight months I was given some of the most toxic substances known to man, poisons that ravaged my body daily. I still felt poisoned—and even now, three years after the fact, I feel that my body isn't quite rid of it yet.

I had absolutely nothing to hide, and the drug tests proved it. It was no coincidence that every time Tour officials chose a rider from our team for random drug testing, I was their man. Drug testing was the most demeaning aspect of the Tour: right after I finished a stage I was whisked to an open tent, where I sat in a chair while a doctor wrapped a piece of rubber tubing around my arm, jabbed me with a needle, and drew blood. As I lay there, a battery of photographers flashed their cameras at me. We called the doctors the Vampires. "Here come the Vampires," we'd say. But the drugs tests became my best friend, because they proved I was clean. I had been tested and checked, and retested.

In front of the media, I said, "My life and my illness and my career are open." As far as I was concerned, that should have been the end of it. There was nothing mysterious about my ride at Sestrière: I had worked for it. I was lean, motivated, and prepared. Sestrière was a good climb for me. The gradient suited me, and so did the conditions—cold, wet, and rainy. If there was something unusual in my performance that day, it was the sense of out-of-body effortlessness I rode with— and that I attributed to sheer exultation in being alive to make the climb. But the press didn't back off, and I decided to take a couple of days off from talking to them.

Meanwhile, the U.S. Postal team was a blue express-train. We entered the transition stages between the Alps and the Pyrenees, riding through an area called the Massif Central. It was odd terrain, not mountainous but hardly flat, either, just constantly undulating so that your legs never got a rest. The roads were lined with waving fields of sunflowers as we turned south toward the Pyrenees.

It was brutal riding; all we did was roll up and down the hills, under constant attack. There was never a place on the route to coast and recover, and riders came at us from all directions. Somehow, we kept most of them in check and controlled the peloton, but the days were broiling and full of tension. It was so hot that in places the road tar melted under our wheels.

Frankie, George, Christian, Kevin, and Peter worked the hardest. Frankie would start the rolling climbs, setting a strong tempo and dropping riders. When Frankie got tired, George would pull, and a few more riders would fall by the wayside, unable to keep our pace. Then came Tyler, who would pick up the pace, dropping even more of our competitors. Finally, I would be left with Kevin, pulling me through the steeps. In that way we whittled down the field.

Each day, the attacks continued. The other riders still felt we were vulnerable, and they were determined to wear us out. We reached a section called the Homme Mort, the Dead Man's Climb, a series of undulations that lasted for miles. The breakaways were constant, and our guys were falling apart: Peter Meinert-Neilsen's knee was sore, Kevin was sick as a dog from the temperature changes in the Alps, and Frankie and George were blown from carrying the load. Everybody's feet hurt, because they swelled in our bike shoes in all that heat.

All of a sudden 30 guys sprinted up the road, and we had to chase them down. It was a flash of my old self—I took off. I didn't wait for Tyler or Frankie or anybody. I just went. I caught up to them, and rode at the front, alone. Then the radio crackled, and I heard Kevin's voice yelling at me. "Goddammit, what are you doing?" I had fallen back into my oldest bad habit, a senseless charge and waste of energy. "Just back off," Kevin warned me. "You don't need to do that."

I sat up and said, "Okay," and I faded back, to conserve myself, while the other Postal riders did the chasing.

What did I think about on the bike for six and seven hours? I get that question all the time, and it's not a very exciting answer. I thought about cycling. My mind didn't wander. I didn't daydream. I thought about the techniques of the various stages. I told myself over and over that this was the kind of race in which I had to always push if I wanted to stay ahead. I worried about my lead. I kept a close watch on my competitors, in case one of them tried a breakaway. I stayed alert to what was around me, wary of a crash.

For five monotonous days and nights, we rode through Central France toward the Pyrenees, from Saint-Etienne to Saint-Galmier to Saint-Flour to Albi to Castres to Saint-Gaudens. Stage 13 was the longest of the tour, and the hottest, with seven climbs and no flats. Frankie said the route profile looked like the edge of a saw blade, and that's what it felt like. Peter Meinert-Neilsen finally abandoned with his bad knee. Some of the hotels were so tiny, Frankie complained that when he sat on the toilet, his knees hit the bathroom door. George claimed that he and Frankie, who were rooming together, couldn't open their suitcases at the same time.

On the bike, we were always hungry and thirsty. We snacked on cookies, tarts, almond cakes, oatmeal-raisin cookies, nutrition bars, any kind of simple carbohydrate. We gulped sugary thirst-quenching drinks, Cytomax during the day and Metabol at the end of it.

At night over our training-table meals, we talked trash, pure junk, embellishing old tales and bragging about conquests, 99 percent of it untrue. We delighted in the storytelling of our chef, Willy Balmet, a 65-year-old Swiss and a dear friend who has cooked for every team I've been on. Willy looks like a much younger man, and can speak six languages, everything short of Swahili. The kitchen was his domain, and in all the years I've known him, I've never once seen him be denied the kitchen in a hotel. He would arrive and make the hotel staff feel a part of our team. He always cooked our pasta; nobody else was allowed to touch it.

While I rode, Kik lit candles all over Europe. No matter what village or metropolis she was in, she would find a church and light a candle. In Rome, she lit one at the Vatican.

FINALLY, WE REACHED THE PYRENEES.

We rode into Saint-Gaudens in the shade of the mountains, through a countryside by Van Gogh. The Pyrenees would be the last chance for the climbers to unseat me: one bad day in those mountains and the race could be lost. I wouldn't be convinced I could win the Tour de France until we came down from the mountains.

The pressure was mounting steadily. I knew what it was like to ride with the pack in 55th place and finish a Tour de France, but the yellow jersey was a new experience and a different kind of pressure. When you're in the yellow jersey, as I was learning, you catch a lot of wind. My fellow riders tested me on the bike every single day. I was tested off the bike, too, as the scrutiny I underwent in the press intensified.

I decided to address the charges outright, and held a press conference in Saint-Gaudens. "I have been on my deathbed, and I am not stupid," I said. Everyone knew that use of EPO and steroids by healthy people can cause blood disorders and strokes. What's more, I told the press, it wasn't so shocking that I won Sestrière; I was an established former world champion.

"I can emphatically say I am not on drugs," I said. "I thought a rider with my history and my health situation wouldn't be such a surprise. I'm not a new rider. I know there's been looking, and prying, and digging, but you're not going to find anything. There's nothing to find . . . and once everyone has done their due diligence and realizes they need to be professional and can't print a lot of crap, they'll realize they're dealing with a clean guy."

All I could do was continue to ride, take drug tests, and deal with the questions. We embarked on the first stage in the Pyrenees, from Saint-Gaudens to Piau-Engaly, a route through seven mountains. This was the same terrain I had ridden when it was so cold, but now as we traveled over col after craggy col it was dusty and hot, and riders begged each other for water. The descents were steep and menacing, with drop-offs along the side of the road.

The stage would finish just over the border from Spain, which meant that all the Spanish riders were determined to win it—and none more than Escartin, the lean, hawk-faced racer who followed me everywhere. In the midst of the frenetic action, our Postal group got separated and I wound up alone, pursuing Escartin. He rode like an animal. All I could hope to do was limit how much time he made up.

As the mountains parted in front of me on the second-to-last climb of the day, I managed to ride Zulle off my wheel and move into second place. But there was no catching Escartin, who had a two-minute gap. On the last climb, I was worn out and I bonked. I hadn't eaten anything solid since breakfast. I got dropped by the leaders and finished fourth. Escartin won the stage and vaulted into second place overall, trailing me by 6:19. Zulle was 7:26 back.

Not long after I crossed the finish line, a French TV journalist confronted me: there were reports that I had tested positive for a banned substance. The report was wrong, of course. I returned to the team hotel, and pushed through a throng of clamoring media, and called another press conference. All I could do was assert my innocence each time there was a new wave of speculation in the papers—and there was one every three or four days.

Le Monde had published a story stating that a drug test had turned up minute traces of corticosteroid in my urine. I was using a cortisone cream to treat a case of saddle sores—and I had cleared the cream with the Tour authorities before the race ever started. Immediately, Tour authorities issued a statement affirming my innocence. *"Le Monde* was looking for a drug story, and they got one on skin cream," I said.

I was hurt and demoralized by the constant barrage from the press. I put forth such effort, and had paid such a high price to ride again, and now that effort was being devalued. I tried to deal with the reports honestly and straightforwardly, but it didn't seem to do any good.

I began to notice something. The people who whispered and wrote that I was using drugs were the very same ones who, when I was sick, had said, "He's finished. He'll never race again." They were the same ones who, when I wanted to come back, said, "No, we don't want to give him a chance. He'll never amount to anything."

Now that I was in the lead of the Tour de France, wearing the yellow jersey, and looking more and more like the eventual winner, the very same people sent the very same message. "It's not possible," they said. "Can't be done. He can't do it. What's going on here? There must be another explanation, something suspicious." They were consistent, the naysayers.

It's a good thing I didn't listen to them when I was sick.

It hurt me, too, that the French journalists in particular were so suspicious of me. I lived in France, and I loved the country. After the previous year's problems during the Tour, a number of top riders had stayed away from France in '99, but not me. While other riders were afraid of being harassed by the police or investigated by the governmental authorities, I trained there every day. France was the most severe place in the world to be caught using a performance enhancer, but I did all of my springtime racing in France, and conducted my entire Tour preparation there. Under French law, the local police could have raided my house whenever they wanted. They didn't have to ask, or knock. They could have sorted through my drawers, rifled my pockets, searched my car, whatever they wanted, without a warrant or any sort of notice.

I said to the press, "I live in France. I spent the entire months of May and June in France, racing and training. If I was trying to hide something, I'd have been in another country."

But they didn't write that, or print that.

The next day, we traveled to perhaps the most famous mountain in the Tour, the Col du Tourmalet. The road to the top soared more than ten miles into the sky. It was our last big climb and test, and once again, we knew we would be under relentless attack. By now we were sick of riding in front, always catching the wind, while being chased from behind. But if we could control the mountains for one more day, it would be hard to deny us the top spot on the podium in Paris.

As soon as we reached the base of the 20-kilometer Tourmalet, the other riders began nipping at us. We rode a strong tempo, trying to weaken the attackers, and with 8K to go, we accelerated. The French climber, Virenque, drew even with Kevin and said, angrily, "What's your problem?" Kevin said he didn't have a problem. Virenque asked Kevin if he was going *"à bloc,"* which means all-out. Kevin said, "No, are you going *à bloc?"* With that, Kevin kicked into a bigger gear and sped away from him. For the rest of the day Virenque chased us, glowering.

As we labored upward, Escartin and I shadowed each other. I watched him carefully. On the steepest part of the climb, he attacked. I went right with him—and so did Zulle. Going over the top it was the three of us, locked in our private race. At the peak, we looked down on a thick carpet of clouds below us. As we descended, the fog closed in and we couldn't see ten feet in front of us. It was frightening, a high-speed chase through the mist, along cliff roads with no guardrails.

All I cared about now was keeping my main rivals either with me or behind me. Ahead of us loomed a second climb, the Col du Soulor. Escartin attacked again, and again I went right with him. We reached another fog-cloaked summit, and now just one more climb remained in the Tour de France: the Col d'Aubisque, 7.5 kilometers of uphill effort. Then the mountain work would be over, and it was an all-out drop to the finish at speeds of up to 70 miles per hour.

There were now three riders in front, fighting for the stage win, and a pack of nine trailing a minute behind and still in contention for the stage, among them myself, Escartin, and Zulle. I didn't care about a stage win. With four kilometers to go, I decided to ride safely and let the rest of them sprint-duel, while I avoided crashes. I had just one aim, to protect the yellow jersey.

I cycled through the stage finish and dismounted, thoroughly exhausted but pleased to have protected my lead. But after five hours on the bike, I now had to face another two-hour press conference. I was beginning to feel that the press was trying to break me mentally, because the other riders couldn't do it physically. The media had become as much of an obstacle as the terrain itself.

That day, the International Cycling Union released all of my drug tests, which were, in fact, clean. What's more, I had received a wonderful vote of confidence from the race organizer, Jean-Marie Leblanc. "Armstrong beating his illness is a sign that the Tour can beat its own illness," he said.

Somehow, we had fended off all the attacks, both on the bike and off, and kept the yellow jersey on my back. We had done it, we had controlled the mountains, and after three weeks and 2,200 miles I led the race with an overall time of 86:46:20. In second, trailing by six minutes and 15 seconds, was Escartin, and in third place, trailing by seven minutes and 28 seconds, was Alex Zulle.

I still wore the *maillot jaune.*

ODDLY, AS PARIS DREW CLOSER, I GOT MORE AND MORE nervous. I was waking up every night in a cold sweat, and I began to wonder if I was sick. The night sweats were more severe than anything I'd had when I was ill. I tried to tell myself the fight for my life was a lot more important than my fight to win the Tour de France, but by now they seemed to be one and the same to me.

I wasn't the only nervous member of our team. Our head mechanic was so edgy that he slept with my bike in his hotel room. He didn't want to leave it in the van, where it could be prey for sabotage. Who knew what freakish things could happen to keep me from winning? At the end of Stage 17, a long flat ride to Bordeaux, some nutcase shot pepper spray into the peloton, and a handful of riders had to pull over, vomiting.

There was a very real threat that could still prevent me from the winning the Tour: a crash. I faced one last obstacle, an individual time trial over 35.4 miles in the theme-park town of Futuroscope. In a time trial very, very bad things could happen. I could fall and break a collarbone, or a leg.

I wanted to win the time trial. I wanted to make a final statement on the bike, to show the press and cycling rumormongers that I didn't care what they said about me. I was through with press conferences (although not with drug tests; I was random-tested yet again after stage 17). To try to win the time trial, however, was a risky proposition, because a rider seeking the fastest time is prone to taking foolish chances and hurting himself—perhaps so badly that he can't get back on the bike.

We saw it all the time. Just look at what happened to Bobby Julich in Metz, when he crashed at 55 mph and suffered massive hematomas in his chest. I'd nearly crashed myself in that time trial, when the child jumped out in front of me as I came around the tight turn. On the Alpe d'Huez, the spectator had jumped in front of Guerini and he crashed. Zulle would have been only a minute behind me if he hadn't crashed on the Passage du Gois.

Bill Stapleton came to see me in the hotel the night before the stage. "Lance, I'm not a coach, but I think you should take it easy here," he said. "You've got a lot to lose. Let's just get through it. Don't do anything stupid."

The smart play was to avoid any mistakes, don't fall, don't hurt yourself, and don't lose ten minutes because of a crash.

I didn't care.

"Bill, who in the fuck do you think you're talking to?" I said.

"What?"

"I'm going to kick ass tomorrow. I'm giving it everything. I'm going to put my signature on this Tour."

"Okay," Bill said, with resignation. "So I guess that's not up for discussion."

I'd worn the yellow jersey since Metz, and I didn't want to give it up. As a team we had ridden to perfection, but now I wanted to win as an individual. Only three riders had ever swept all of the time trials in the Tour, and they happened to be the three greatest ever:

Bernard Hinault, Eddy Merckx, and Miguel Indurain. I wanted to be among them. I wanted to prove I was the strongest man in the race.

I couldn't sleep. Scott MacEachern from Nike came back to my room to visit, and so did Stapleton. Johan stuck his head in the room and saw Scott sprawled on my bed, while I was still on my feet. Johan looked at his watch: it was 11:30 P.M. "Get these guys out of here and go to bed," he ordered me.

My mother flew in for Futuroscope, and I arranged for her to ride in one of the follow cars. She wanted to see the time trial because she felt that old protective instinct; if she was with me, I wouldn't get hurt. But the time trials frightened her as much as anything, because she understood cycling well enough to know how easily I could crash—and she knew this day, the second-to-last of the race, would either make it or break it for me, once and for all. She had to be there for that.

A time trial is a simple matter of one man alone against the clock. The course would require roughly an hour and 15 minutes of riding flat-out over 57 kilometers, a big loop through west-central France, over roads lined with red tiled roofs and farm fields of brown and gold grass, where spectators camped out on couches and lounge chairs. I wouldn't see much of the scenery, though, because I would be in a tight aerodynamic tuck most of the time.

The riders departed in reverse order, which meant I would be last. To prepare, I got on my bike on a stationary roller, and went through all the gears I anticipated using on the course.

While I warmed up, Tyler Hamilton had his go at the distance. His job was to ride as hard and fast as he could, regardless of risk, and send back technical information that might help me. Tyler not only rode it fast, he led for much of the day. Finally, Zulle came in at 1 hour, 8 minutes, and 26 seconds to knock Tyler out of first place.

It was my turn. I shot out of the start area and streaked through the

winding streets. Ahead of me was Escartin, who had started three minutes before I did.

My head down, I whirred by him through a stretch of trees and
long grass, so focused on my own race that I never even glanced at
him.

I had the fastest time at the first two splits. I was going so fast that
in the follow car, my mother's head jerked back from the acceleration
around the curves.

After the third time check I was still in first place at 50:55. The
question was, could I hold the pace on the final portion of the race?

Going into the final six kilometers, I was 20 seconds up over Zulle.
But now I started to pay. I paid for mountains, I paid for the undulations, I paid for the flats. I was losing time, and I could feel it. If I beat
Zulle, it would be only by a matter of seconds. Through two last,
sweeping curves, I stood up. I accelerated around the corners, trying
to be careful not to crash, but still taking them as tightly as I could—
and almost jumped a curb and went up on the pavement.

I raced along a highway in the final sprint. I bared my teeth, counting, driving. I crossed the line. I checked the time: 1:08:17.

I won by 9 seconds.

I cruised into a gated area, braked, and fell off the bike, bent over
double.

I had won the stage, and I had won the Tour de France. I was now
assured of it. My closest competitor was Zulle, who trailed in the overall standings by 7 minutes and 37 seconds, an impossible margin to
make up on the final stage into Paris.

I was near the end of the journey. But there had been two journeys,
really: the journey to get to the Tour, and then the journey of the Tour
itself. In the beginning there was the Prologue and the emotional
high, and that first week, uneventful but safe. Then there were the
strange out-of-body experiences at Metz and Sestrière, followed by the

demoralizing attacks by the press. Now to finish with a victory gave me a sweet sense of justification. I was going to Paris wearing the *maillot jaune.*

As I took the podium my mother clapped and waved a flag and wiped her eyes. I hadn't seen her before the stage, but immediately afterward I grabbed her in a hug, and then took her to lunch. She said, "You're just not going to believe what's going on back home. I know it's hard for you to understand or even think about right now. But the people in the U.S. are going crazy. I've never seen anything like this before."

Afterward, we went back to the hotel, and another throng of press was in the lobby. We worked our way through the crowd toward my room, and one of the French journalists tried to interview my mother. "Can we talk?" he asked.

I turned around and said: "She's not speaking to the French press." But the guy continued to ask her a question.

"Leave her alone," I said. I got my arm around her and steered us through the crowd up to my room.

THAT NIGHT, I BEGAN TO GET AN IDEA OF THE RE-sponse back home in the States. A journalist from *People* magazine arrived and wanted an interview. Sponsors streamed into our team hotel to shake hands and visit. Friends began to arrive; they had jumped on planes overnight. Bill Stapleton took me to dinner and explained that all of the morning shows and late-night talk shows wanted me to appear. He thought I should fly to the States for a day after the Tour for a series of TV interviews.

But traditionally, the Tour winner travels to a series of races around Europe to display the yellow jersey, and I wanted to honor that. "It's not up for discussion," I said. "I'm staying here to do these races."

"Okay, fine," Bill said. "Great."

"Well, what do you think?"

"I think you're being really stupid."

"Why?"

"Because you have no idea what's going on back there, and how important it is. But you're going to find out. The day this thing is over, you cannot hide. Everybody in America is paying attention."

Nike wanted me to hold a press conference in New York at their mega-store, and the mayor wanted to be there, and so did Donald Trump. The people in Austin wanted to have a parade. Nike offered a private jet to fly me to the States and back to Europe in a single day, so I could do the races. I was stunned. I'd spent years winning bike races, and nobody in the States had cared.

Now everybody cared.

But part of me still didn't entirely trust the fact that I was going to win. I told myself there was one more day to race, and after dinner I stayed sequestered, got my hydration and my rubdown, and went to bed.

The final stage, from Arpajon into Paris, is a largely ceremonial ride of 89.2 miles. According to tradition, the peloton would cruise at a leisurely pace, until we saw the Eiffel Tower and reached the Arc de Triomphe, where the U.S. Postal team would ride at the front onto the Champs-Elysées. Then a sprint would begin, and we would race ten laps around a circuit in the center of the city. Finally, there would be a post-race procession, a victory lap.

As we rode toward Paris, I did interviews from my bike and chatted with teammates and friends in the peloton. I even ate an ice-cream cone. The Postal team, as usual, rode in superbly organized fashion. "I don't have to do anything," I said to one TV crew. "It's all my boys."

After a while another crew came by. "I'd like to say Hi to Kelly Davidson, back in Fort Worth, Texas," I said. "This is for you." Kelly is the young cancer fighter who I'd met in the Ride for the Roses, and she and her family had become my close friends.

Finally, we approached the city. I felt a swell of emotion as we rode onto the Champs-Elysées for the first time. The entire avenue was shut down for us, and it was a stunning sight, with hundreds of thousands of spectators lining the avenue of fitted cobblestones and brick. The air was full of air horns and confetti, and bunting hung from every facade. The number of American flags swirling in the crowd stunned me.

Deep in the crowd, someone held up a large cardboard sign. It said "TEXAS."

As we continued to parade down the Champs, it gradually dawned on me that not all of those flags were the Stars and Stripes. Some of those waving pennants, I saw delightedly, were from the Lone Star State.

The ten-lap sprint to the finish was oddly subdued and anticlimactic, a formality during which I simply avoided a last freak crash. And then I crossed the finish line. It was finally tangible and real. I was the winner.

I dismounted into pandemonium; there were photographers everywhere, and security personnel, and protocol officials, and friends, clapping me on the back. There must have been 50 people from Austin, including Bart Knaggs, and my dear friend Jeff Garvey, and even, believe it or not, Jim Hoyt. Homeboy had talked his way into our compound.

I was ushered to the podium for the victory ceremony, where I raised the trophy after it was presented to me. I couldn't contain myself anymore, and leaped down and ran into the stands to embrace my wife. The photographers surrounded me, and I said, "Where's my Mom?" and the crowd opened and I saw her and grabbed her in a hug. The press swarmed around her too, and someone asked her if she thought my victory was against the odds.

"Lance's whole life has been against all odds," my mother told him.

Then came the best part of all, the ceremonial victory lap where I rode with the team one last time. We cruised all alone on the Champs-Elysées. We had been together for three weeks, and we rode very, very slowly, savoring the moment. A stranger dashed into the street and handed me a huge American flag on a pole. I don't know how he got there—he just appeared in front of me and thrust it into my hand. I raised the flag, feeling an overwhelming blur of sensation and emotion.

Finally, I returned to the finish area and spoke to the press, choking back tears. "I'm in shock. I'm in shock. I'm in shock," I said. "I would just like to say one thing. If you ever get a second chance in life for something, you've got to go all the way."

We were whisked away as a team, to get ready for that night's celebration banquet, an elaborate fête for 250 people at the Musée d'Orsay, surrounded by some of the most priceless art in the world. We were exhausted to a man, utterly depleted by the three-week ordeal, but we looked forward to raising a glass.

We arrived at the museum to find the tables exquisitely set, except for the rather odd centerpieces, which had been suggested by Thom Weisel.

There was an arrangement of apples at each place.

We lifted our first glasses of Champagne since Metz, and I stood to toast my teammates. "I wore the yellow jersey," I said. "But I figure maybe the only thing that belongs to me is the zipper. A small piece of it. My teammates deserve the rest—sleeves, the front and back of it."

My teammates raised their hands.

There was something clenched in the fist of each man.

An apple. Red, shiny apples, all around me.

THAT NIGHT, KRISTIN AND I CHECKED INTO THE RITZ, where we'd booked a huge and expensive suite. We changed into the complimentary bathrobes and opened another bottle of Champagne, and had our private moment, our celebration. We were finally alone together again, and we giggled at the size of the suite, and had dinner from room service. Then we fell into a very deep sleep.

I woke up the next morning and burrowed down into the pillow, and tried to adjust to the unfamiliar surroundings. Next to me, Kik opened her eyes, and gradually we came fully awake. As she stared at me, we read each other's thoughts.

"Oh, my God," I said. *"I won the Tour de France."*

"No way," she said.

We burst out laughing.

ten

THE CEREAL BOX

THE TRUTH IS, IF YOU ASKED ME TO CHOOSE between winning the Tour de France and cancer, I would choose cancer. Odd as it sounds, I would rather have the title of cancer survivor than winner of the Tour, because of what it has done for me as a human being, a man, a husband, a son, and a father.

In those first days after crossing the finish line in Paris I was swept up in a wave of attention, and as I struggled to keep things in perspective, I asked myself why my victory had such a profound effect on people. Maybe it's because illness is universal—we've all been sick, no one is immune—and so my winning the Tour was a symbolic act, proof that you can not only survive cancer, but thrive after it. Maybe, as my friend Phil Knight says, I am hope.

Bill Stapleton finally convinced me that I needed to fly to New York for a day. Nike provided the private jet, and Kik came with me, and in New York, the full reach and impact of the victory finally hit us. I had a press conference at Niketown, and the mayor did show up, and so did Donald Trump, and I appeared on the *Today* show, and on David Letterman. I went to Wall Street to ring the opening bell. As I walked onto the trading floor, the traders erupted in sustained applause, stunning me. Then, as we left the building, I saw a huge throng of people gathered on the sidewalk. I said to Bill, "I wonder what that crowd is doing here?"

"That's for you, Lance," Bill said. "Are you starting to get it now?"

Afterward, Kik and I went to Babies "Я" Us. People came down the aisles of the store to shake my hand and ask for autographs. I was taken aback, but Kik was unfazed. She just said, blithely, "I think we need some onesies and a diaper pail."

To us, there was a more ordinary act of survival still to come: parenthood.

AT FIRST, I WORRIED THAT BECAUSE I DIDN'T HAVE A relationship with my own father, I might not make a good one myself.

I tried to practice being a father. I bought a sling to carry the baby in, and I wore it around the house, empty. I strapped it on and wore it in the kitchen while I made breakfast. I kept it on when I sat in my office, answering mail and returning phone calls. I strolled in the backyard with it on, imagining that a small figure was nestled there.

Kik and I went to the hospital for a tour of the facilities and a nurse briefed us on what to expect when Kik went into labor.

"After the baby is delivered it will be placed on Kristin's chest," she said. "Then we will cut the umbilical cord."

"I'll cut the umbilical cord," I said.

"All right," the nurse said agreeably. "Next, a nurse will bathe the baby . . ."

"*I'll* bathe the baby."

"Fine," the nurse said. "After that, we will carry the baby down the hall . . ."

"*I'll* carry the baby," I said. "It's my baby."

One afternoon late in her pregnancy, Kik and I were running errands in separate cars, and I ended up tailgating her home. I thought she was driving too fast, so I dialed her number on the car phone.

"Slow it down," I said. "That's my child you're carrying."

In those last few weeks of her pregnancy, Kik liked to tell people, "I'm expecting my *second* child."

In early October, about two weeks before the baby was due, Bill Stapleton and I went to Las Vegas, where I was to deliver a speech and hold a couple of business meetings. When I called home, Kik told me she was sweating and felt strange, but I didn't think much about it at first. I went on with my business, and when I was done, Bill and I dashed to catch an afternoon flight back to Dallas, with an evening connection to Austin.

In a private lounge area in Dallas I called Kik, and she said she was still sweating, and now she was having contractions.

"Come on," I said. "You're not really having this baby, are you? It's probably a false alarm."

On the other end of the line, Kik said, "Lance, this is not funny."

Then she went into a contraction.

"Okay, okay," I said. "I'm on my way."

We boarded the plane for Austin, and as we took our seats, Stapleton said, "Let me give you a little marital advice. I don't know if your wife's having a baby tonight, but we need to call her again when we get up in the air."

The plane began its taxi, but I was too impatient to wait for take-off, so I called her from the runway on my cell phone.

"Look, what's going on?" I said.

"My contractions are a minute long, and they're five minutes apart, and they're getting longer," she said.

"Kik, do you think we're having this baby tonight?"

"Yeah, I think we're having the baby tonight."

"I'll call you as soon as we land."

I hung up, and ordered two beers from the flight attendant, and Bill and I clinked bottles and toasted the baby. It was just a 40-minute flight to Austin, but my leg jiggled the whole way there. As soon as landed, I called her again. Usually, when Kik answers the phone she says "Hi!" with a voice full of enthusiasm. But this time she picked up with a dull "Hi."

"How you feeling, babe?" I said, trying to sound calm.

"Not good."

"How we doing?"

"Hold on," she said.

She had another contraction. After a minute she got back on.

"Have you called the doctor?" I said.

"Yeah."

"What'd he say?"

"He said to come into the hospital as soon as you get home."

"Okay," I said. "I'll be there."

I floored it. I drove 105 in a 35 zone. I screeched into the driveway, helped Kik into the car, and then drove more carefully to St. David's Hospital, the same place where I had my cancer surgery.

Forget what they tell you about the miracle of childbirth, and how it's the greatest thing that ever happens to you. It was horrible, terrifying, one of the worst nights of my life, because I was so worried for Kik, and for our baby, for all of us.

Kik had been in labor for three hours as it turned out, and when the delivery-room staff took a look at her and told me how dilated she was, I told her, "You're a stud." What's more, the baby was turned "sunny side up," with its face toward her tailbone, so she had racking pains in her back.

The baby was coming butt-first, and Kik had trouble delivering. She tore, and she bled, and then the doctor said, "We're going to have to use the vacuum." They brought out something that practically looked like a bathroom plunger, and they attached it to my wife. They performed a procedure, and—and the baby popped right out. It was a boy. Luke David Armstrong was officially born.

When they pulled him out he was tiny, and blue, and covered with birth fluids. They placed him on Kik's chest, and we huddled together. But he wasn't crying. He just made a couple of small, mew-like sounds. The delivery-room staff seemed concerned that he wasn't making more noise. *Cry,* I thought. Another moment passed, and still Luke didn't cry. *Come on, cry.* I could feel the room grow tense around me.

"He's going to need a little help," someone said.

They took him away from us.

A nurse whisked the baby out of Kik's arms and around a corner into another room, full of complicated equipment.

Suddenly, people were running.

"What's wrong?" Kik said. "What's happening?"

"I don't know," I said.

Medical personnel dashed in and out of the room, as if it was an emergency. I held Kik's hand and I craned my neck, trying to see what was going on in the next room. I couldn't see our baby. I didn't know what to do. My son was in there, but I didn't want to leave Kik, who was terrified. She kept saying to me, "What's going on, what are they doing to him?" Finally, I let go of her hand and peered around the corner.

They had him on oxygen, with a tiny mask over his face.

Cry, please. Please, please cry.

I was petrified. At that moment I would have done anything just to hear him scream, absolutely anything. Whatever I knew about fear was completely eclipsed in that delivery room. I was scared when I was diagnosed with cancer, and I was scared when I was being treated, but it was nothing compared to what I felt when they took our baby away from us. I felt totally helpless, because this time it wasn't me who was sick, it was somebody else. It was my son.

They removed the mask. He opened his mouth, and scrunched his face, and all of a sudden he let out a big, strong "Whaaaaaaaaaa!!!" He screamed like a world-class, champion screamer. With that, his color changed, and everyone seemed to relax. They brought him back to us. I held him, and I kissed him.

I bathed him, and the nurse showed me how to swaddle him, and together, Kik and Luke and I went to a large hospital room that was almost like a hotel suite. It had the regulation hospital bed and equipment, but it also had a sofa and a coffee table for visitors. We slept together for a few hours, and then everyone began to arrive. My mother came, and Kik's parents, and Bill and Laura Stapleton. That first evening, we had a pizza party. Visitors stuck their heads in our door to see Kik sitting up in bed sipping a Shiner Bock and chewing on a slice.

My mother and I took a stroll through the corridors, and I couldn't help thinking about what I had just gone through with Luke. I completely understood now what she must have felt when it seemed as though she might outlive her own child.

We passed by my old hospital room. "Remember that?" I asked. We smiled at each other.

THE QUESTION THAT LINGERS IS, HOW MUCH WAS I A factor in my own survival, and how much was science, and how much miracle?

I don't have the answer to that question. Other people look to me for the answer, I know. But if I could answer it, we would have the cure for cancer, and what's more, we would fathom the true meaning of our existences. I can deliver motivation, inspiration, hope, courage, and counsel, but I can't answer the unknowable. Personally, I don't need to try. I'm content with simply being alive to enjoy the mystery.

Good joke:

A man is caught in a flood, and as the water rises he climbs to the roof of his house and waits to be rescued. A guy in a motorboat comes by, and he says, "Hop in, I'll save you."

"No, thanks," the man on the rooftop says. "My Lord will save me."

But the floodwaters keep rising. A few minutes later, a rescue plane flies overhead and the pilot drops a line.

"No, thanks," the man on the rooftop says. "My Lord will save me."

But the floodwaters rise ever higher, and finally, they overflow the roof and the man drowns.

When he gets to heaven, he confronts God.

"My Lord, why didn't you save me?" he implores.

"You idiot," God says. "I sent you a boat, I sent you a plane."

I think in a way we are all just like the guy on the rooftop. Things take place, there is a confluence of events and circumstances, and we can't always know their purpose, or even if there is one. But we *can* take responsibility for ourselves and be brave.

We each cope differently with the specter of our deaths. Some people deny it. Some pray. Some numb themselves with tequila. I was tempted to do a little of each of those things. But I think we are supposed to try to face it straightforwardly, armed with nothing but courage. The definition of courage is: the quality of spirit that enables one to encounter danger with firmness and without fear.

It's a fact that children with cancer have higher cure rates than adults with cancer, and I wonder if the reason is their natural, unthinking bravery. Sometimes little kids seem better equipped to deal with cancer than grown-ups are. They're very determined little characters, and you don't have to give them big pep talks. Adults know too much about failure; they're more cynical and resigned and fearful. Kids say, "I want to play. Hurry up, and make me better." That's all they want.

When Wheaties decided to put me on the cover of the box after the Tour de France, I asked if we could hold the press conference in the children's cancer ward at the same hospital where my son was born. As I visited with the kids and signed some autographs, one little boy grabbed a Wheaties box and stood at my knees, clutching it to his chest.

"Can I have this?" he said.

"Yeah, you can have it," I said. "It's yours."

He just stood there, looking at the box, and then he looked back at me. I figured he was pretty impressed.

Then he said, "What shapes are they?"

"What?" I said.

"What *shapes* are they?"

"Well," I said, "it's *cereal*. It's all different shapes."

"Oh," he said. "Okay."

See, to him, it's not about cancer. It's just about cereal.

IF CHILDREN HAVE THE ABILITY TO IGNORE ODDS AND percentages, then maybe we can all learn from them. When you think about it, what other choice is there but to hope? We have two options, medically and emotionally: give up, or fight like hell.

After I was well again, I asked Dr. Nichols what my chances really were. "You were in bad shape," he said. He told me I was one of the worst cases he had seen. I asked, "How bad was I? Worst fifty percent?" He shook his head. "Worst twenty percent?" He shook his head again. "Worst ten?" He still shook his head.

When I got to three percent, he started nodding.

Anything's possible. You can be told you have a 90-percent chance or a 50-percent chance or a 1-percent chance, but you have to believe, and you have to fight. By fight I mean arm yourself with all the available information, get second opinions, third opinions, and fourth opinions. Understand what has invaded your body, and what the possible cures are. It's another fact of cancer that the more informed and empowered patient has a better chance of long-term survival.

What if I had lost? What if I relapsed and the cancer came back? I still believe I would have gained something in the struggle, because in what time I had left I would have been a more complete, compassionate, and intelligent man, and therefore more alive. The one thing the illness has convinced me of beyond all doubt—more than any experience I've had as an athlete—is that we are much better than we know. We have unrealized capacities that sometimes only emerge in crisis.

So if there is a purpose to the suffering that is cancer, I think it must be this: it's meant to improve us.

I am very firm in my belief that cancer is not a form of death. I choose to redefine it: it is a part of life. One afternoon when I was in remission and sitting around waiting to find out if the cancer would come back, I made an acronym out of the word: Courage, Attitude, Never give up, Curability, Enlightenment, and Remembrance of my fellow patients.

In one of our talks, I asked Dr. Nichols why he chose oncology, a field so difficult and heartbreaking. "Maybe for some of the same reasons you do what you do," he said. In a way, he suggested, cancer is the Tour de France of illnesses.

"The burden of cancer is enormous, but what greater challenge can you ask?" he said. "There's no question it's disheartening and sad, but even when you don't cure people, you're always helping them. If you're not able to treat them successfully, at least you can help them manage the illness. You connect with people. There are more human moments in oncology than any other field I could imagine. You never get used to it, but you come to appreciate how people deal with it—how strong they are."

"You don't know it yet, but we're the lucky ones," my fellow cancer patient had written.

I will always carry the lesson of cancer with me, and feel that I'm a member of the cancer community. I believe I have an obligation to make something better out of my life than before, and to help my fellow human beings who are dealing with the disease. It's a community of shared experience. Anyone who has heard the words *You have cancer* and thought, "Oh, my God, I'm going to die," is a member of it. If you've ever belonged, you never leave.

So when the world seems unpromising and gray, and human nature mean, I take out my driver's license and I stare at the picture, and I think about LaTrice Haney, Scott Shapiro, Craig Nichols, Lawrence Einhorn, and the little boy who likes cereal for their shapes. I think about my son, the embodiment of my second life, who gives me a purpose apart from myself.

Sometimes, I wake up in the middle of the night and I miss him. I lift him out of his crib and I take him back to bed with me, and I lay him on my chest. Every cry of his delights me. He throws back his tiny head and his chin trembles and his hands claw the air, and he wails. It sounds like the wail of life to me. "Yeah, that's right," I urge him. "Go on."

The louder he cries, the more I smile.